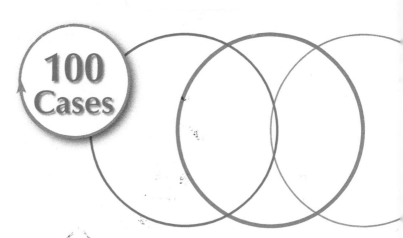

100 Cases

in Emergency Medicine and Critical Care

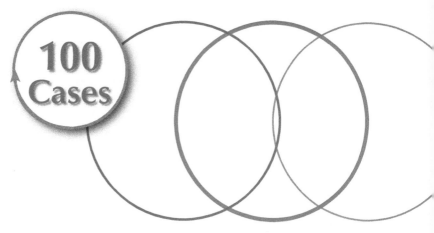

in Emergency Medicine and Critical Care

Eamon Shamil MBBS MRes MRCS DOHNS, AFHEA
Specialist Registrar in ENT – Head & Neck Surgery
Guy's and St Thomas' NHS Foundation Trust, London, UK

Praful Ravi MA MB BChir MRCP
Resident in Internal Medicine, Mayo Clinic, Rochester, MN, USA

Dipak Mistry MBBS BSc DTM&H FRCEM
Consultant in Emergency Medicine, University College London
Hospital NHS Foundation Trust, London, UK

100 Cases Series Editor:
Janice Rymer
Professor of Obstetrics & Gynaecology and Dean of Student Affairs,
King's College London School of Medicine, London, UK

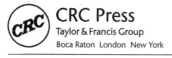

CRC Press
Taylor & Francis Group
Boca Raton London New York

CRC Press is an imprint of the
Taylor & Francis Group, an **informa** business

CRC Press
Taylor & Francis Group
6000 Broken Sound Parkway NW, Suite 300
Boca Raton, FL 33487-2742

Printed on acid-free paper
Printed by CPI Group (UK) Ltd, Croydon CR0 4YY

International Standard Book Number-13: 978-1-139-03547-8 (Paperback)
International Standard Book Number-13: 978-1-138-57253-9 (Hardback)

Visit the Taylor & Francis Web site at
http://www.taylorandfrancis.com

and the CRC Press Web site at
http://www.crcpress.com

CONTENTS

Mental Health and Overdose

Neurology and Neurosurgery

Trauma and Orthopaedics

General Surgery and Urology

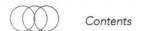

Medicolegal

CONTRIBUTORS

Mental Health and Overdose, Ophthalmology, Maxillofacial

Dr Mohsan M. Malik BSc, MBBS
Specialist Trainee in Ophthalmology
The Royal London Hospital
Barts Health NHS Trust
London, UK

Obstetrics and Gynaecology

Dr Hannan Al-Lamee MPhil, MBChB
Specialist Trainee in Obstetric and Gynaecology
Imperial College Healthcare NHS Trust
London, UK

Paediatrics

Dr Noor Kafil-Hussain BSc, MBBS, MRCPCH
Specialist Trainee in Paediatric Medicine
London Deanery
London, UK

Neurology and Neurosurgery

Dr Vin Shen Ban MB BChir, MRCS, MSc, AFHEA
Resident in Neurological Surgery
University of Texas Southwestern Medical School
Dallas, Texas

INTRODUCTION

Emergency Medicine and Critical Care are difficult specialties and they can be quite daunting for new physicians. The modern Emergency Medicine physician has to take a focused history, which can often be incomplete due to the patient's care being spread over several hospitals, examining the patient, arranging rational investigations and then treating the patient. This is often combined with seeing multiple patients simultaneously as well as time pressure. Similarly, in Critical Care, there is the challenge of having to very rapidly assess unwell or deteriorating patients and initiating a suitable management strategy.

This book has been written for medical students, doctors and nurse practitioners. One of the best methods of learning is case-based learning. This book presents a hundred such 'cases' or 'patients' which have been arranged by system. Each case has been written to stand alone so that you may dip in and out or read sections at a time.

Detail on treatment has been deliberately rationalised as the focus of each case is to recognise the initial presentation, the underlying pathophysiology, and to understand broad treatment principles. We would encourage you to look at your local guidelines and to use each case as a springboard for further reading.

We hope that this book will make your experience of Emergency Medicine and Critical Care more enjoyable and provide you with a solid foundation in the safe management of patients in this setting, an essential component of any career choice in medicine.

Eamon Shamil
Praful Ravi
Dipak Mistry

CRITICAL CARE

History

An 84-year-old patient is brought into the resuscitation area of the Emergency Department by a blue-light ambulance. He is in obvious respiratory distress and has a tracheostomy secondary to advanced laryngeal cancer.

Examination

On examination, he is cyanotic and visibly tired with a respiratory rate of 28. His oxygen saturation is 84% on room air, blood pressure 94/51, pulse 120 and temperature 36.4°C.

Questions

1. What are the indications for a tracheostomy?
2. How do you manage a patient with a tracheostomy in respiratory distress?
3. What is the standard care for a tracheostomy patient?

DISCUSSION

A tracheostomy refers to a stoma between the skin and the trachea. It means that air bypasses the upper aerodigestive tract. This removes the natural mechanisms of voice production (larynx) and humidification (nasal cavity). Patients are more prone to chest infections from mucus accumulating in the lungs.

Tracheostomy emergencies may be encountered in the Emergency Department, Intensive Care Unit or the ward.

Indications for a tracheostomy include the following:

- Weaning patients from prolonged mechanical ventilation is the commonest indication in ICU. The tracheostomy reduces dead space and the work of breathing compared to an endotracheal tube. The TracMan study in the United Kingdom has shown that there is no difference in hospital length of stay, antibiotic use or mortality between early (day 1–4 ICU admission) or late (day 10 or later) tracheostomy.
- Emergency airway compromise – e.g. supraglottitis, laryngeal neoplasm, vocal cord palsy, trauma, foreign body, oedema from burns and severe anaphylaxis.
- In preparation for major head and neck surgery.
- To manage excess trachea–bronchial secretions – e.g. in neuromuscular disorders where cough and swallow is impaired.

If a patient with a tracheostomy is in respiratory distress

Call for urgent help from both an anaesthetist and an ENT surgeon and have a difficult airway trolley at the bedside. Apply oxygen (15 L/min) via a non-rebreather mask to the face and tracheostomy site. Use humidified oxygen if available. Look, listen and feel for breathing at the mouth and tracheostomy site. Remove the speaking valve and inner tracheostomy tube, and then insert a suction catheter to remove secretions that may be causing the blockage. If suction does not help, deflate the tracheostomy cuff so air can pass from the mouth into the lungs. Look, listen and feel for breathing and use waveform capnography to monitor end-tidal CO_2. If the patient is not improving and is NOT in imminent danger, then a fibreoptic endoscope can be inserted into the tracheostomy to inspect for displacement or obstruction.

If a single lumen tracheostomy is blocked and suction and cuff deflation does not provide adequate ventilation, remove the tracheostomy and insert a new tube of the same or smaller size whilst holding the stoma open with tracheal dilators. If you cannot insert a new tracheostomy tube, insert a bougie into the stoma or railroad a tube over a fibreoptic endoscope to allow insertion under direct vision.

If you are unable to unblock or change the tracheostomy tube, then perform bag-valve mask ventilation via the nose and mouth with a deflated tracheostomy cuff and cover stoma with gauze and tape to prevent air leak. If this does not work, then try to bag-valve-mask ventilate over the tracheostomy stoma after closing the patient's mouth and nose. If the patient has normal anatomy (i.e. no airway obstruction from a tumour or infection), then think about oral intubation or bougie-guided stoma intubation.

In contrast, laryngectomy patients have an end stoma and cannot be oxygenated by the mouth or nose unlike tracheostomy patients. If passing a suction catheter does not unblock a laryngectomy tube/stoma, then remove the laryngectomy tube from the stoma and look, listen and feel or apply waveform capnography to assess patency. If the stoma is not patent, apply a paediatric facemask to the stoma and ventilate. A secondary attempt can be made to intubate the laryngectomy stoma with a small tracheostomy tube or cuffed endotracheal tube. A fibre-optic endoscope can be used to railroad the endotracheal tube in the correct position.

Post-tracheostomy care should be conducted by an appropriately trained nurse or trained patient/carer and includes

- Humidified oxygen with regular suctioning
- Bedside spare tracheostomy tube, introducer and tracheal dilators
- Pen and paper for patient to communicate
- Tracheostomy change after 7 days to allow speaking valve application and formation of a stoma tract
- Patient and family education

 Key Points

- Indications for a tracheostomy include the following: weaning patients from prolonged mechanical ventilation, emergency airway compromise, in preparation for major head and neck surgery and managing excess trachea–bronchial secretions
- When facing a tracheostomy patient in respiratory distress, think of the three C's:
    1. Cuff – Put the cuff down so the patient can breathe around it.
    2. Cannula – Change the inner cannula.
    3. Catheter – Insert a suction catheter into the tracheostomy.

History

A 54-year-old man has been admitted into the Intensive Care Unit with severe gallstone pancreatitis, complicated by acute kidney injury and acute respiratory distress syndrome (ARDS). He is currently intubated and ventilated, and requires haemofiltration. He will likely require a prolonged hospital admission.

The intensive care consultant asks you to 'take care of his nutrition'.

Questions

1. What are the causes of nutritional disturbance?
2. How can nutrition be assessed?
3. What are the options for optimising nutrition? Name some complications.

DISCUSSION

Nutrition is an important part of every patient's care and should be optimised with the help of a dietician, in parallel with treating his or her underlying pathology. It should be assessed soon after admission as it is estimated that around a quarter of hospital inpatients are inadequately nourished. This may be due to increased nutritional requirements (e.g. in sepsis or post-operatively), nutritional losses (e.g. malabsorption, vomiting, diarrhoea) or reduced intake (e.g. sedated patients).

Signs of malnutrition include a body mass index (BMI) under 20 kg/m², dehydration, reduced tricep skin fold (fat) and indices such as reduced mid-arm circumference (lean muscle) or grip strength. Low serum albumin is sometimes quoted as a marker of malnutrition, but this is not an accurate marker in the early stages as it has a long half-life and may be affected by other factors including stress.

The body's predominant sources of energy are fat (approximately 9.3 kcal/g of energy), glucose (4.1 kcal/g) and protein (4.1 kcal/g). The recommended daily intake of protein is around 1 g/kg; nitrogen 0.15 g/kg; calories 30 kcal/kg/day. A patient's basal energy expenditure is doubled in head injuries and burns. The major nutrient of the small bowel is amino acid glutamine, which improves the intestinal barrier thereby reducing microbe entry. The fatty acid butyrate is the major source of energy for cells of the large bowel (colonocytes).

There are two options for nutrition, namely enteral (through the gut) and parenteral (intravenous). Enteral feeding can be administered by different routes including oral, nasogastric (NG) tube, nasojejunal (NJ) tube and percutaneous endoscopic gastrostomy (PEG)/jejunostomy (PEJ). Enteral nutrition is generally preferred to parenteral nutrition as it keeps the gut barrier healthy, reduces bacterial translocation and has less electrolyte and glucose disturbances. Feeding through the mouth is the ideal scenario as it is safe and provides adequate nutrition. Before abandoning oral intake, patients should be tested on semi-solid or puree diets and reassessed for risk of aspiration (e.g. in stroke).

When comparing NG and NJ tube feeding, NG tubes are advantageous in terms of being larger in diameter and less likely to block, whereas NJ tubes are better if a patient is at risk of lung aspiration as they bypass the stomach. NJ tubes are also used in pancreatitis as they bypass the duodenum and pancreatic duct, which reduces pancreatic enzyme release that would have exacerbated pancreatic inflammation. NG/NJ feeds should be built up gradually, and if the patient experiences diarrhoea or distention, the feed can be slowed down. Patients on a feed should undergo initially daily blood tests for re-feeding syndrome, which causes deficiencies in potassium, phosphate and magnesium.

Total parenteral nutrition (TPN) is composed of lipids (30% of calories), protein (20% of calories) and carbohydrates (50% of calories in the form of dextrose), as well as water, electrolytes, vitamins and minerals. TPN is indicated in patients who have inadequate gastrointestinal absorption (short bowel syndrome), or where bowel rest is needed (e.g. gastrointestinal fistula or bowel obstruction). The disadvantage of TPN compared to enteral nutrition is that it is more expensive, contributes to gut atrophy if prolonged and exacerbates the acute phase response. Other complications of TPN include intravenous line infection or insertion complication, re-feeding syndrome, fatty liver, electrolyte and glucose imbalance and acalculous cholecystitis.

🔑	Key Points

- Nutrition should be optimised in all patients, in parallel with treating their underlying pathology. A dietician should be involved especially where critical care input or prolonged inpatient stay is predicted.
- There are two types of nutrition, enteral and parenteral. If it is safe and provides adequate nutrition, oral intake is the preferred option.
- NG/NJ/TPN feeding all have complications including re-feeding syndrome, which can cause hypophosphatemia, hypokalaemia and hypomagnesaemia.

History

A 48-year-old man presents with shortness of breath, painful swallowing and hoarseness. This is on a background of a worsening sore throat for the past 3 days. He has not been on antibiotics.

The patient experiences sore throats several times per year, but never this severe. He does not have any other medical problems and does not take regular medications. He doesn't smoke or drink alcohol, and he works in the supermarket, but has been off work since yesterday.

Examination

There is obvious inspiratory stridor heard from the end of the bed. The patient is sitting upright with an extended neck on the edge of the bed. He is drooling, sweating and struggling to speak. His vital signs are as follows: temperature of 38.8°C, respiratory rate of 28, oxygen saturation of 96% on room air, pulse of 107 beats per minute, blood pressure of 100/64 mmHg.

He has bilateral non-tender cervical lymphadenopathy. His oropharynx demonstrates bilaterally enlarged grade 3 tonsils with white exudate. There is pooled saliva in the oral cavity. Flexible fibreoptic naso-pharyngo-laryngoscopy demonstrates a normal nasal cavity and nasopharynx. However, there is marked inflammation of the supraglottis including a cherry-coloured epiglottis and oedematous aryepiglottic folds. The vocal cords are not swollen and fully mobile.

Questions

1. What is the diagnosis?
2. What investigations are appropriate?
3. How would you manage this patient? Which teams would you involve, and what is the major concern?

DISCUSSION

This patient has supraglottitis. This is a life-threatening emergency with risk of upper airway obstruction. This is caused by an infection of the supraglottis, which is the upper part of the larynx, above the vocal cords, including the epiglottis.

It is important to appreciate that halving the radius of the airway will increase its resistance by 16 times (Poiseuille's equation), and hearing stridor means there is around 75% airway obstruction.

Supraglottitis, which includes acute epiglottitis, is bimodal, with presentations most common in children under 10 years old and adults between 40 and 50 years old. Classically the causative organism in children is *Haemophilus influenzae* type B, but since the advent of its vaccination, the incidence has reduced in children. The infection is now twice as common in adults, even if they have been vaccinated. The most common organisms are now Group A *Streptococcus*, *Staphylococcus aureus*, *Klebsiella pneumoniae* and beta-haemolytic *Streptococci*. Viruses such as HSV-1 and fungi including candida are an important cause in immunocompromised patients.

Sore throat and odynophagia occur in the majority of patients. Other signs include drooling, dysphonia, fever, dyspnoea and stridor. In adults, the disease has more of a gradual onset, with a background of sore throat for 1–2 days, whereas in children, the disease progresses more acutely.

In children, the disease may be confused with croup (laryngotracheobronchitis). To distinguish these clinically, epiglottitis tends to be associated with drooling, whereas croup has a predominant cough. Other diagnoses to consider in adults and children include tonsillitis, deep neck space infection, such as retro- or para-pharyngeal abscess, and foreign body in the upper aerodigestive tract. In adults, an advanced laryngeal cancer may also have a similar presentation.

Investigations such as venepuncture and examination of the mouth should be deferred in children, as upsetting the child may precipitate airway obstruction. Adults are more tolerant to investigations and should include an arterial blood gas, intravenous cannulation and drawing of blood for blood cultures, a full blood count and electrolyte testing. Radiographic imaging including x-rays should be avoided in the acute setting. The use of bedside naso-pharyngo-laryngoscopy allows direct visualization of the pathology.

This patient should be initially assessed and managed in the resuscitation area by a senior emergency medicine doctor. After a quick assessment, prompt involvement of a multidisciplinary team should take place. This should include a senior anaesthetist, ENT surgeon and intensive care doctors.

Airway resuscitation and temporizing measures include the following:
- Sit upright.
- 15 L/min oxygen via a non-rebreather mask to keep oxygen saturations above 94%.
- Nebulised adrenaline (5 mL 1:1000) to reduce tissue oedema and inflammation.
- IV or intramuscular corticosteroids (e.g. 8 mg dexamethasone IV) to reduce tissue oedema and inflammation.
- Broad-spectrum IV antibiotics as per local microbiology guidelines (e.g. ceftriaxone and metronidazole) to combat the infective process.

- Ensure there is an emergency airway trolley at the bedside including a needle crico-thyroidotomy and surgical cricothyroidotomy set.
- If there is Heliox, ask for it (79% helium, 21% oxygen) as this has a lower density and higher laminar flow than air, which can buy time in an acute scenario.

A joint anaesthetic–ENT airway assessment should take place in an area with access to emergency airway resuscitation equipment, ideally in the operating theatre. This should include fibreoptic flexible nasopharyngo-laryngoscopy. The patient should be warned of the possibility of a tracheostomy and ideally sign a written consent form prior to any intervention.

A discussion should take place between all members of the team to plan for possible complications. Best practice would be to have the ENT surgeon scrubbed and ready to perform an emergency tracheostomy while the anaesthetist attempts intubation either under direct vision or by video laryngoscopy/fibreoptic scopes. If this fails, an ENT surgeon may attempt rigid bronchoscopy, surgical cricothyroidotomy or tracheostomy.

If intubation is likely to fail due to the amount of airway obstruction and poor visualization of the glottis, then a local anaesthetic tracheostomy should be performed.

Management of epiglottitis in children differs. Oxygen or nebulisers may be wafted over their mouth, but IV antibiotics and steroids should be deferred if they may upset the child. The priority is to transfer the child, accompanied by a parent, to the operating theatre for assessment and management.

Postoperatively, the patient should be managed in the intensive care unit with regular IV antibiotics and steroids. After around 48 hours, extubation may be attempted if there are signs of improvement. Daily assessment of the supraglottic area should take place with flexible nasendoscopy.

 Key Points

- Supraglottitis is a life-threatening airway emergency that usually presents with odynophagia, dysphonia and dyspnoea on the background of a sore throat. It can affect children and adults.
- Multidisciplinary management in the resuscitation area of the Emergency Department or in theatres is required. The team should include an emergency physician, anaesthetist, ENT surgeon and an intensivist.
- Emergency airway management prior to definitive control by endotracheal intubation or tracheostomy should include 15 L/min oxygen through non-rebreather mask, nebulised adrenaline, intravenous steroids and broad-spectrum antibiotics.

CASE 4: COLLAPSE WHILE HIKING

History

A 55-year-old man is brought to the Emergency Department after collapsing while hiking with his son. Bystander CPR was performed for 5 minutes before the paramedics arrived and continued resuscitation. The rhythm was ventricular fibrillation (VF), and a total of 8 shocks were delivered before return of spontaneous circulation. He has a history of hypertension and type 2 diabetes, controlled with medications. He is a smoker, but there is no family history of sudden cardiac death.

Examination

Vital signs: temperature of 37.5°C, blood pressure of 105/55, heart rate of 95 and regular.

He is intubated, ventilated and sedated with fentanyl and propofol. Physical examination is notable for normal heart sounds and bilateral breath sounds. GCS is 3/15.

 Investigations

- Hb 14.6, WCC 15.3, PLT 275, Cr 95.
- Arterial blood gas: pH 7.15 pO_2 22.5, pCO_2 4, HCO_3 20, lactate 7.5.
- A chest radiograph shows appropriate positioning of the endotracheal tube. An ECG shows Q waves in the anterior leads.

Questions

1. Describe the general principles of post-resuscitation care. Should therapeutic hypothermia be initiated?
2. Is there any role for coronary revascularisation (i.e. angiography) in this patient?
3. How can this patient's prognosis be assessed?

DISCUSSION

This patient presents with an out of hospital cardiac arrest (OHCA) with successful resuscitation after a relatively prolonged period. The main aims of management in OHCA are to minimise secondary neurologic injury, to appropriately support cardiac function and to look for a cause.

Post-resuscitation care should proceed along an 'ABCDE' approach, and since most patients will have a low Glasgow Coma Score, the airway should be protected with intubation and mechanical ventilation as has occurred in this case. In addition to assessing for signs of circulatory shock (cool peripheries, mottled skin), it is also important to look for signs that are suggestive of the underlying cause (e.g. heart murmur, rigid abdomen). A basic neurologic assessment to calculate the GCS pre-intubation is necessary as this correlates with neurologic outcomes and provides a baseline for future comparison.

Key initial investigations that should be performed include an electrocardiogram (to look for cardiac ischaemia), bedside ultrasonography (looking for pulmonary embolism, assess for ventricular function, fluid status or abdominal aortic aneurysm) and a chest radiograph. Additional blood tests, including an arterial blood gas and renal function, are important as they may point towards the underlying cause. D-dimer and troponin will often be elevated and need careful evaluation in the clinical context.

Current recommendations state that patients with shockable OHCA should be cooled to prevent secondary brain injury. This is termed therapeutic hypothermia. It is suggested that patients with non-shockable OHCA are cooled too. Core body temperature should be lowered to between 32 and 36°C by removing clothes and infusing cooled saline or by using external cooling jackets. The aim is to reduce secondary brain injury by decreasing cellular metabolism.

The role for coronary angiography in OHCA has not been completely defined, and there is variation in practice across treatment centres. Emergent coronary angiography is indicated in patients with ECG findings of ST elevation myocardial infarction (i.e. ST elevation, new left bundle branch block) and is typically performed urgently in patients in whom a cardiac cause is suspected. In this patient, given the presence of a VF arrest and anterior Q-waves on the electrocardiogram, you should liaise with the local cardiology service. In large cities, patients may be taken directly to cardiology centres bypassing the ED in patients with a VF/VT arrest and return of spontaneous circulation (ROSC).

After successful resuscitation from an OHCA, only 10% of patients will survive to discharge, and many of these individuals will have significant neurologic disability. Prognostication is difficult, but negative prognostic factors include delayed initiation of CPR, PEA or asystolic arrests, older age and persistent coma. Absent corneal or pupillary reflexes at 24 hours, absent visual evoked potentials and elevated serum neuron-specific enolase (NSE) are poor prognostic markers.

Key Points
• Out of hospital cardiac arrest is an important and common cause of mortality in developed countries.
• Post-resuscitation care should proceed in an 'ABCDE' manner, with the aim to minimise brain injury and support cardiac function.
• Therapeutic hypothermia is recommended for all patients with a shockable OHCA and suggested for non-shockable cases.
• Coronary angiography and reperfusion therapy should be considered in those patients thought to have an underlying cardiac cause.
• Prognosis after out of hospital cardiac arrest is generally poor.

History

A 20-year-old student is brought to the Emergency Department after his room-mate noticed that he did not attend a class tutorial and found him in a semi-conscious state. He had been feeling generally unwell for the past 2–3 days after fresher's week and complained of a headache. He has no other past medical history and only takes anti-histamines as needed for hayfever.

Examination

Vital signs: temperature of 39.4°C, heart rate of 100 and regular, blood pressure of 95/60, respiratory rate of 16, 95% O_2 saturation on air.

Physical examination reveals a pale man who intermittently follows commands. GCS is 12/15 (Eyes 3, Verbal 4, Motor 5). There is a purpuric rash on his arms and legs, and bleeding from his gums. Neurologic examination is notable for neck stiffness. Cardiorespiratory examination is unremarkable.

Questions

1. What is the diagnosis, and what complication is the patient likely suffering from?
2. What investigations need to be performed immediately?
3. What empiric treatment should the patient receive in the Emergency Department?

DISCUSSION

This patient presents with fever, reduced level of consciousness and evidence of meningism on examination, which are classic for bacterial meningitis. This is a condition that is fatal unless promptly recognised and treated. The two most common pathogens causing bacterial meningitis are *Streptococcus pneumoniae* and *Neisseria meningitidis*. In this patient, the latter is the likely cause due to the presence of the petechial rash seen with meningococcal disease; additionally, bleeding from the gums suggests disseminated intravascular coagulation (DIC), which is associated with meningococcal sepsis.

Meningococcal meningitis has a high mortality, with 10%–15% of patients dying of the disease despite appropriate therapy. Therefore, the role of the Emergency Department physician is crucial in initiating treatment. Sick patients should be assessed and treated along the standard 'ABCDE' approach, and antibiotics given early after drawing baseline blood tests and blood cultures. Ceftriaxone and vancomycin will provide broad spectrum cover and are first-line empiric therapy. If the diagnosis is uncertain and encephalitis is suspected, add an antiviral agent (i.e. aciclovir).

Aside from antibiotics, good supportive care with intravenous fluid and vasopressors as well as supplemental titrated oxygen is key. There is no specific treatment for DIC except treating the underlying infection, although there is limited evidence that protein C concentrate may improve coagulopathy but not mortality. Dexamethasone has been shown to be beneficial in pneumococcal meningitis by reducing neurological complications but has no clear benefit in meningococcal infection.

A lumbar puncture should be performed after a CT head. CSF fluid analysis may show organisms such as Gram-negative diplococci (*Neisseria meningitidis*), and the white cell count will be elevated (neutrophilic predominance) together with elevated CSF protein and low CSF glucose. PCR studies may be performed to give a rapid diagnosis of the causative organism.

Another key aspect of managing this patient involves gathering a history of contact exposure as antibiotic prophylaxis is required in close contacts ('kissing contacts'). Anyone with prolonged (i.e. >8 hours) and close contact with the patient as well as those directly exposed to the patient's oral secretions will need chemoprophylaxis. The choice of agent may vary according to local guidelines, but a single dose of either ciprofloxacin, rifampicin or ceftriaxone is commonly used. The public health department will need to be informed in confirmed meningitis cases as it is a 'notifiable' disease and can help with contact tracing and prophylaxis.

 Key Points

- Patients presenting a fever and headache should be considered at risk for meningitis.
- Meningococcal meningitis is a rapidly fatal disease and must be recognised and treated promptly.
- Empiric antibiotic therapy for suspected meningitis comprises of ceftriaxone and vancomycin, and blood and cerebrospinal fluid cultures should be obtained to help tailor therapy towards the pathogen.
- The public health department must be contacted as this is a 'notifiable' disease.

History

A 27-year-old man presents to the Emergency Department with a 1-day history of nausea, vomiting and feeling generally unwell. He reports pain over his right lower leg and some redness overlying the area. He has a history of type 1 diabetes and is on a 'basal-bolus' regime comprising of daily glargine and mealtime novorapid. He does not check his blood sugars frequently and does not recall when he last took insulin.

Examination

Vital signs: temperature of 37.6°C, blood pressure of 90/60, heart rate of 100 and regular, respiratory rate of 24, 96% O_2 saturation on air.

His peripheries are cool and capillary refill time is 2 s; JVP is not visible and mucous membranes are dry. Cardiorespiratory examination is unremarkable and abdominal palpation reveals generalised tenderness. There is an erythematous area on his right shin with associated warmth and tenderness to touch. Neurologic examination is normal.

Investigations
• Hb 15.6, WCC 16.7 (neutrophils 13.5), PLT 210, Na 132, K 3.4, Cl 98, Ur 11.5, Cr 80.
• Venous blood gas shows: pH 7.15, pO_2 12.4, pCO_2 4.1, HCO_3 16, glucose 28, lactate 4.7.

Questions

1. What is the diagnosis, and the likely precipitating factor in this case?
2. What further investigations should be performed in the Emergency Department?
3. What are the initial steps in the management of this patient? How should the patient be monitored?

DISCUSSION

The most important diagnosis to exclude in any patient with type 1 diabetes who is unwell is diabetic ketoacidosis (DKA), whereby insulin deficiency leads to impaired glucose utilisation by cells and the production of ketone bodies leading to a metabolic acidosis. DKA usually develops over a 24-hour period, and the symptoms seen in this patient (nausea and vomiting) are a common manifestation. Additionally, the elevated respiratory rate seen is likely a compensatory response to metabolic acidosis (Kussmaul breathing). Common precipitating factors in DKA include infection, lack of compliance with insulin therapy and intercurrent illness. Infection and acute illness promote a stress response with production of counter-regulatory hormones (e.g. glucagon, adrenaline) and lead to relative insulin deficiency. In this case, the patient appears to be suffering from a concurrent right leg cellulitis.

The initial evaluation of DKA includes measuring electrolytes, serum glucose and a venous blood gas. Additionally, urinalysis should be performed to look for urine ketones – many centres can also measure serum ketones to confirm the diagnosis. An electrocardiogram should be performed given the presence of mild hypokalaemia in this patient. Further investigations should be directed at identifying the potential precipitating cause (e.g. chest radiograph and urine culture, swab of any purulent material expressed from the leg). It would also be reasonable to check an HbA$_1$C if none has been performed recently to determine glycaemic control.

DKA is a medical emergency and carries a low, but not insignificant, mortality risk. Initial assessment and management should follow the standard 'ABCDE' approach. The first step in treating DKA is to replace the fluid deficit, which can be up to several litres. This patient shows signs of hypovolaemic shock and therefore 1 L boluses of isotonic fluid (0.9% saline) should be given with monitoring of haemodynamic response. Once his blood pressure improves and tachycardia settles, fluid replacement should continue as per local protocol, normally as a reducing regime of intravenous fluid. Potassium replacement is required given that insulin therapy will lead to intracellular movement of potassium out of the vascular space, with 20–30 mmol added to each litre of saline administered.

Intravenous insulin (actrapid) is the second major component of DKA treatment and serves to turn off the ketogenic switch. It should be commenced at a fixed rate of 0.1 units/kg/hour, equating to 7 units/hour in a 70 kg individual. Adjunctive therapy in DKA includes administration of bicarbonate (typically only if pH < 6.9), although there is limited evidence for its benefit, as well as treatment of the underlying cause (e.g. antibiotics for cellulitis).

Once initial treatment is begun, patients require careful monitoring, ideally in a high dependency care setting. The rate of fluid administration needs to be tailored according to haemodynamic parameters, and serum glucose and potassium should be checked frequently (hourly to begin with). Once glucose falls to below 10–12 mmol/L, the rate of the insulin infusion may be reduced, although each hospital may have its own protocol. Venous (or arterial) pH should also be checked regularly together with urine or serum ketones, as the resolution of ketoacidosis is an indicator that subcutaneous insulin can be commenced, providing the patient can eat, with overlap of intravenous insulin for 1–2 hours.

Patients with a low GCS and who do not show immediate improvement with initial resuscitation should have a CT scan of the head to look for cerebral oedema. They may need intubation to protect their airway and for ventilatory control prior to scan. Cerebral oedema is more commonly seen in children but may also occur in adults. The aetiology is not clear but it may be related to severely acidotic states and fluid shifts associated with rehydration.

 Key Points

- Always consider diabetic ketoacidosis (DKA) in any diabetic patient who is unwell.
- Check serum electrolytes, glucose, urine ketones and serum ketones, as well as a venous blood gas in patients with suspected DKA.
- Fluid replacement, potassium repletion and intravenous insulin are the mainstays of the early management of DKA.

History

A 17-year-old man is brought to the Emergency Department by his mother after he was stung by an insect. He had been playing football at the local park when his mother thought she saw a bee near his leg. He is feeling nauseous and reports a rash on his leg that is spreading to the rest of his body. He complains that his throat feels itchy and feels like he is having palpitations. He has a history of asthma.

Examination

Vital signs: temperature of 36.8°C, blood pressure of 85/60, heart rate of 110 and regular, respiratory rate of 24, 95% O$_2$ saturation on air.

General examination reveals a blotchy, erythematous rash on his right leg that is spreading upwards towards his trunk, as well as swelling of his lips and tongue. Cardiac examination is unremarkable, and auscultation of the chest is notable for mild expiratory wheeze.

Questions

1. What is the diagnosis? Briefly describe its pathophysiology.
2. How would you manage the patient?
3. Assuming he responds appropriately to treatment, does the patient need to be admitted? Is any follow-up required?

DISCUSSION

This patient is suffering from anaphylaxis, which is an acute-onset potentially life-threatening allergic or hypersensitivity reaction. The diagnosis of anaphylaxis can be made when *any one* of the following is present:

i. Acute onset illness that involves the skin and/or mucosa, with either respiratory compromise or hypotension
ii. Two or more of the following that occur quickly after exposure to a known allergen for a patient: involvement of the skin/mucosa, hypotension, respiratory compromise or persistent gastrointestinal symptoms
iii. Hypotension after exposure to a known allergen for a patient (defined as systolic BP <90 mm Hg in adults, or ≥30% decrease from baseline)

In this case, there is no history of an allergic reaction, but the patient has skin/mucosal involvement (widespread rash), respiratory difficulty (tachypnoea, presence of wheeze) and hypotension, thereby meeting the first criterion for diagnosis of anaphylaxis. The majority of cases are mediated by a type I hypersensitivity reaction, where pre-formed allergen-specific IgE (produced from prior sensitisation) on mast cells and basophils interacts with the allergen, resulting in degranulation and release of chemokines such as histamine.

Anaphylaxis is a medical emergency and must be quickly recognised and treated. Management should proceed along the 'ABCDE' approach; the airway should be secured first and preparations for intubation made should there be evidence of stridor or significant tongue/pharyngeal oedema. Supplemental oxygen should be delivered to maintain saturations >94% and large-bore intravenous cannulae placed, along with initiation of a fluid bolus.

The most important treatment in anaphylaxis is adrenaline. The normal dose is 0.5 mg (0.5 mL of 1:1000 solution) in adults, and it is usually administered intramuscularly into the outer thigh. The dose may be repeated at an interval of 3–5 minutes should there be no response.

Adjunctive treatments include bronchodilators (salbutamol 5 mg nebulised), anti-histamines (chlorpheniramine 10 mg IV) and steroids (hydrocortisone 200 mg IV), as well as fluid boluses titrated to blood pressure. In non-responders, intravenous adrenaline may be given in 50 μg boluses, but this should only be given by senior ED, anaesthetic or intensive care physicians due to the danger of precipitating cardiac ischaemia. Take care to remove the suspected source of anaphylaxis if possible such as a retained insect sting as in this case or other potential sources like colloid solution or blood products.

Anyone who has had a severe reaction or required multiple doses of adrenaline should be admitted for observation for a biphasic reaction. Those with a single dose of adrenaline may be discharged after 6 hours if they are symptom free. At discharge, patients should be prescribed an adrenaline auto-injector ('Epipen', usual dose 0.3 mg) and consider once daily oral prednisolone for up to 3 days. Follow-up should also be arranged with an allergy specialist, who may arrange further testing to identify the allergen and initiate preventive therapy.

UK guidelines suggest mast cell tryptase should be measured on arrival and subsequent samples at 2 and 12 hours. It may be particularly helpful when patients suffer from an allergic reaction in unusual circumstances (e.g. when under general anaesthetic) or to confirm the diagnosis when features are atypical such as isolated angioedema. Blood testing should not, however, delay treatment, which should be based on clinical grounds.

Key Points

- Always think of anaphylaxis when seeing patients with skin/mucosal symptoms, respiratory difficulty and/or hypotension, especially after exposure to a potential allergen.
- Adrenaline 0.5 mg IM is the first-line treatment.
- Any patient with an anaphylactic reaction must at least be observed for several hours in case of biphasic reaction, and any patient with a severe reaction should be admitted.

CASE 8: A BAD CHEST INFECTION

History

A 55-year-old man presents with a 3-day history of a productive cough and shortness of breath. He has a history of chronic obstructive pulmonary disease (COPD) with frequent exacerbations but no previous intensive care admissions. He is a current smoker and type 2 diabetic, and takes inhaled tiotropium and subcutaneous glargine daily.

Examination

Vital signs: weight of 90 kg, temperature of 38.5°C, blood pressure of 85/50, heart rate of 105 and regular, respiratory rate of 25, 94% O_2 saturation on 4 L/min.

Physical examination is notable for coarse crackles and bronchial breathing at the right lower lung fields.

Investigations
• Hb 16, WCC 18.5 (neutrophils 15), PLT 200, Ur 8, Cr 135, lactate 3.5. Blood and sputum cultures are pending.
• A chest radiograph shows opacification of the right base.
• He is given a 500 mL fluid bolus, a urinary catheter is inserted and empiric broad-spectrum antibiotics (vancomycin and piperacillin-tazobactam) are commenced. He is transferred to the Intensive Care Unit (ICU) for further management, where a central line and arterial line are placed.

Questions

1. What would be the initial goals of therapy in the ICU in the first few hours of admission, and what parameters should be monitored to assess response to treatment?
2. After 6 hours, he has received 6 L of intravenous fluid and his blood pressure remains 85/50, urine output is 30 mL/hour and lactate has increased to 4.5. What is the term given to this condition, and outline of the next steps in management?
3. How should his diabetes be managed while he is critically ill?

DISCUSSION

This patient presents with symptoms and signs suggestive of sepsis, likely arising from a chest infection. He is febrile, hypotensive, tachycardic and hypoxic, and has an elevated white blood cell count and lactate, all indicators of a dysregulated inflammatory reaction to infection which defines a sepsis syndrome.

The initial resuscitation provided to the patient is appropriate and is discussed fully in another case ('Dysuria and weakness', Case 18, page 63). The goal of initial resuscitation is to restore perfusion and prevent or limit organ dysfunction. The term 'early goal-directed therapy' (EGDT) refers to the administration of intravenous fluid within the first 6 hours of presentation that uses various physiologic targets to direct fluid management. These targets or goals include

    i.   Mean arterial blood pressure (MAP) ≥65 mmHg
    ii.   Urine output ≥0.5 mL/kg/hour
    iii.   Central venous pressure (CVP) of 8–12 mmHg
    iv.   Central venous oxyhaemoglobin saturation ($ScvO_2$) ≥70%
    v.   Clearance of lactate

While randomised evidence on the benefit of using such targets in a protocol-based manner is conflicting, it is standard practice in most centres. In particular, targeting CVP 8–12 mmHg, MAP ≥65 mmHg and urine output ≥0.5 mL/kg/hour are commonly used in the ICU setting, and achieved via the administration of fluid boluses with continuous measurement of these parameters to ensure that the rate of fluid administration can be adjusted accordingly.

In this case, reassessment after 6 hours reveals that the patient's MAP is 62 mmHg, urine output is <45 mL/hour (he weighs 90 kg) and lactate has increased, suggesting inadequate perfusion. Moreover, these have occurred after plentiful administration of intravenous fluid (1 L/hour), and the presence of refractory hypotension and inadequate perfusion despite seemingly adequate fluid resuscitation is termed septic shock. In this situation, the use of vasopressor and inotropic agents is required.

Remember that MAP is a product of cardiac output (CO) and systemic vascular resistance (SVR). Typically, the first-line vasopressor used in septic shock is noradrenaline, which acts on α_1 and β_1 adrenergic receptors, leading to vasoconstriction (hence increased SVR) and so results in an increase in cardiac output. It is administered via continuous infusion through a central line with the dose adjusted based upon the parameters described above (typically MAP and urine output). If maximal doses of the first vasopressor are inadequate, a second agent such as adrenaline, dobutamine or vasopressin is added.

In addition to achieving haemodynamic stability, it is important to be aware of additional aspects of managing septic shock, which include appropriate management of diabetes and insulin. Hyperglycaemia (blood glucose >10 mmol/L) is associated with poor outcomes and may arise due to the stress response to infection or as a result of coexisting diabetes. In these circumstances, a continuous insulin infusion or intermittent short-acting insulin (e.g. actrapid) is used as they can be adjusted easily and reduce the risk of hypoglycaemia. Generally, a blood glucose target of 7.5–10 mmol/L is used to titrate the insulin infusion rate, as intensive insulin therapy increases the risk of hypoglycaemia, which may lead to increased mortality.

🔑 **Key Points**

- Early goal-directed therapy utilises various physiologic parameters, including MAP ≥65 mmHg and urine output ≥0.5 mL/kg/hour, to guide fluid management within the first 6 hours of a diagnosis of sepsis.
- Septic shock, which is defined by refractory hypotension despite adequate fluid administration, requires the use of vasopressor and inotropic agents such as noradrenaline to maintain perfusion.
- Hyperglycaemia is common in critical illness, particularly in diabetic patients, and is usually managed with a continuous insulin infusion to maintain a blood glucose target of 7.5–10 mmol/L.

History

A 35-year-old male is brought in by ambulance. He was the driver of a vehicle involved in a head-on collision with another vehicle. Both vehicles were travelling at 50 miles per hour and the patient was restrained by a seatbelt.

On arrival to the resuscitation area of the Emergency Department, he is confused and disorientated, unable to confirm his name or age. He is tachypnoeic with a respiratory rate of 32, 97% O_2 saturation on 15 L/min oxygen via a non-rebreather mask, heart rate of 130, blood pressure of 91/49 and temperature of 35.8°C.

In the ambulance, he received 1 L of 0.9% normal saline and 1 unit of Group O Rhesus-negative packed red cells. Despite this, his respiratory rate, heart rate and level of confusion have worsened.

Examination

He is maintaining his airway and is working hard to breathe, with an obvious strap mark on his chest secondary to his seatbelt. His chest expansion is symmetrical with reduced breath sounds in the bases of both lungs. His heart sounds are muffled with marked engorgement of the external jugular veins in the neck. The remainder of his examination is unremarkable with no injury to the head, spine, abdomen or limbs.

A portable chest radiograph shows a possible widened mediastinum, increased cardiac shadow and numerous bilateral rib fractures. The lung fields are opacified bilaterally. The patient's vital signs improve slightly but remain unstable. The patient is taken to theatre for an emergency thoracotomy.

Questions

1. What is the underlying diagnosis?
2. Define shock. What are its signs?
3. How do you manage shock in the haemorrhaging patient?

DISCUSSION

This patient has sustained blunt trauma that has caused cardiac tamponade, bilateral hae-mothoraces and hypovolaemic shock. Shock refers to inadequate organ perfusion and tissue oxygenation. The commonest cause in an injured patient is hypovolaemic shock due to blood loss, but other causes include cardiogenic shock due to myocardial dysfunction, neurogenic shock due to sympathetic dysfunction or obstructive shock due to obstruction of the great vessels or heart.

It is easy to recognise shock if you think about the results of inadequate organ perfusion. Early signs include tachycardia, which is the body's way of attempting to preserve cardiac reserve and cool peripheries or reduced capillary refill time due to peripheral vasocon-striction. This is caused by catecholamine and vasoactive hormone release, which result in increased diastolic blood pressure and reduced pulse pressure. For this reason, measuring pulse pressure rather than systolic blood pressure allows earlier detection of hypovolaemic shock, as the body can lose up to 30% of its blood volume before a drop in systolic blood pressure is appreciated. Brain hypoperfusion initially causes anxiety and later confusion. In summary, tachycardia, cool skin and reduced pulse pressure are early signs of shock until proven otherwise.

It is important to realise that large volumes of blood loss may only cause a minimal drop in haemoglobin or haematocrit levels in the acute setting. More commonly, you will see an elevated lactate level and negative base excess on the venous blood gas, which corresponds to vasoconstriction and cellular hypoxia. Do not wait for a trauma patient to develop hypo-tension before starting fluid replacement therapy. The goal is to maintain organ perfusion and tissue oxygenation. Start with a crystalloid fluid bolus of 20 mL/kg for children or 1 L in adults. Ensure the crystalloid fluid is warmed in order to prevent hypothermia. In those who have sustained significant blood loss, consider early transfusion of packed red cells and activation of the major haemorrhage protocol.

Current trauma guidelines suggest that a degree of hypotension may be tolerated in certain circumstances. This is termed 'balanced resuscitation' or 'permissive hypotension'. The prin-ciple behind this is to stabilise any clots that may have formed as these as thought to be the most stable. Aggressive blood pressure rises may risk disrupting the 'first clot' and exacerbate blood loss. This is still a developing field and local guidelines should be followed. In any hypotensive trauma patient, seek senior help early to help guide management as decisions can be complex and experience in this setting is an asset.

To assess response to fluid resuscitation, monitor level of consciousness, improvement in tachycardia and skin temperature or capillary refill time (as mentioned earlier, these are good early signs of shock). Urine output measurement is also a useful marker (>0.5 mL/kg/hour for adults).

The response to initial fluid resuscitation is key to determining subsequent management. Three possibilities exist:

1. The haemodynamically normal patient with adequate tissue oxygenation and nor-mal vital signs after fluid resuscitation. This patient is a rapid responder to fluid therapy and likely lost 10%–20% of their blood volume.
2. The haemodynamically stable patient with improved but persistently abnormal vital signs (tachycardia and oliguria) following fluid therapy. This patient is under-resuscitated and has transiently responded to fluids. Their tissue oxygenation may

respond to further fluid therapy, but if it does not, they will require definitive surgical management. They have likely lost 20%–40% of their blood volume and may lose more.

3. The haemodynamically unstable patient who continues to deteriorate despite aggressive fluid resuscitation. In this scenario, emergency surgical management as well as ongoing blood replacement may be required.

Depending on the urgency of the blood transfusion, the following products are available. Type O Rhesus negative packed red cells are used for the exsanguinating patient, where there is no time to wait for cross-matching. Type-specific blood compatible with ABO and Rhesus blood types takes 10–20 minutes to obtain from the laboratory and is useful for transient responders. Fully cross-matched blood is the most preferable product and takes around 1 hour to obtain from the laboratory.

Aside from administering a blood transfusion (packed red cells), do not neglect transfusing the patient with platelets, fresh frozen plasma and cryoprecipitate. Large volume blood loss consumes coagulation factors and precipitates a coagulopathy in around 30% of severely injured patients. Within 1 hour of presentation, ensure a full clotting screen has performed to allow early detection of these.

The focus of treatment is to identify and treat the cause of bleeding. Adjuncts in the trauma setting include focused assessment sonography in trauma (FAST), as well as radiographic imaging of the chest, pelvis and long bones of the limbs. It is now accepted practice to perform CT scanning from the head to the thigh in a major trauma scenario. This is a fast and accurate way of detecting life-threatening injuries, allowing appropriate medical and surgical intervention. Ensure that the patient is haemodynamically stable before transfer to the CT scanner as transfer times may be prolonged and deterioration whilst en route or in the scanner is difficult to deal with.

 Key Points

- Shock refers to inadequate organ perfusion and tissue oxygenation. Its signs include tachycardia, reduced pulse pressure and cool peripheries.
- Management of hypovolaemic shock should include warm crystalloid fluid resuscitation with early consideration of a blood transfusion to restore the oxygen-carrying capacity of the intravascular volume.
- The cause of the hypovolaemic shock should be identified and addressed whilst resuscitation is ongoing. Ultrasonography, radiographs and CT scanning can be considered if the patient is stable enough.

History

A 48-year-old male was the driver in a head-on collision between two cars travelling at 45 miles per hour. He has an open tibial fracture and a distended and bruised abdomen. During the primary survey in the Emergency Department, it is noted that he is hypotensive and tachycardic.

A decision is made to initiate fluid resuscitation.

Questions

1. What is the content of 0.9% saline and Hartmann's solution?
2. How is water distributed in the body?
3. How is 1 L of crystalloid fluid distributed in the body? How is 1 L of 5% dextrose solution distributed in the body? How is 1 L of blood distributed in the body?

DISCUSSION

Intravenous fluids can be divided into crystalloids and colloids. Crystalloids are made up of water-soluble molecules (e.g. saline solution, Hartmann's solution). Colloid fluids contain insoluble molecules (e.g. Gelofusin, which contains gelatin).

Saline solution (0.9% sodium chloride) contains both sodium (154 mmol/L) and chloride (154 mmol/L). Hartmann's solution contains the following: sodium 131 mmol/L, chloride 111 mmol/L, potassium 5 mmol/L, calcium 2 mmol/L and bicarbonate 29 mmol/L (which is supplied in the form of lactate, which is then metabolised to bicarbonate).

Sixty percent percent of the human body mass is composed of water, of which two-thirds lies in the intracellular compartment and one-third lies in the extracellular compartment. The extracellular compartment is further subdivided into interstitial fluid (75%) and intravascular fluid (25%). Thus, a 70 kg human will have 42 L of total body water (60% of mass), of which 28 L (two-thirds) is intracellular and 14 L (one-third) is extracellular. Of the extracellular water, 10.5 L (75%) is interstitial and 3.5 L (25%) is intravascular fluid.

To calculate what volume of 1 L of crystalloid such as saline 0.9% or Hartmann's solution enters the intravascular space, the above principles apply. The sodium content of both of these fluids is similar to plasma, which means the entire 1 L of fluid will be distributed amongst the extracellular compartment. Thus, 750 mL (75%) will be interstitial, and 250 mL (25%) will be intravascular. Five percent of dextrose or glucose solutions are distributed relative to total body water, so that 666.6 mL is intracellular and 333.3 mL is extracellular. Of the extracellular fluid, 250 mL is interstitial and 83.3 mL is intravascular. Of note, when administering a blood transfusion, all of the content is distributed in the intravascular space, making it ideal for hypotensive resuscitation.

The disadvantage of using colloids such as Gelofusin is that they contain insoluble proteins that can cause bleeding disorders, interfere with blood cross-matching and may lead to anaphylaxis. Although colloids provide more initial intravascular expansion, it is now accepted that there is no significant difference in reducing mortality when using crystalloids or colloids for fluid resuscitation. This was demonstrated in the Saline versus Albumin Fluid Evaluation (SAFE) Study (2004), which showed that albumin (colloid) and saline (crystalloid) should be considered clinically equivalent treatments for intravascular volume resuscitation in a heterogeneous population of patients in the Intensive Care Unit. Further studies on fluid resuscitation of patients with traumatic brain injury have shown that colloids are associated with a higher mortality than crystalloids.

 Key Points

- When resuscitating a hypotensive patient, using 1 L of crystalloid will equate to 250 mL of intravascular fluid; using 1 L of dextrose 5% will equate to less than 100 mL of intravascular fluid; and using 1 L of blood will equate to 1 L of intravascular fluid.
- Advanced Trauma Life Support (ATLS) guidelines and the SAFE study recommend crystalloid instead of colloid fluid resuscitation. Crystalloids are cheaper and do not exhibit the same disadvantages (blood clotting disorders and anaphylaxis) as colloids.

History

A 48-year-old man is brought into the Emergency Department resuscitation area. He was found unconscious in a burning house. The mechanism of the fire and duration of exposure are unknown.

Examination

Assessment reveals a singeing of the nasal hairs, carbon-stained saliva, oropharyngeal oedema and extensive deep partial thickness burns to the face and neck and full thickness burns to the chest and upper limbs. His oxygen saturation is 88% on air, with a respiratory rate of 22 with limited chest expansion, pulse of 107, blood pressure – no reading obtainable.

Questions

1. How do you classify thermal burns?
2. How would you manage this patient?
3. What are the concerns when it comes to electrical burns?

DISCUSSION

This patient has severe thermal burns and is at high risk of complications of smoke inhalation. These include airway obstruction, restrictive chest expansion, carbon monoxide poisoning, hypovolaemic shock (as burns cause increased capillary permeability and loss of intravascular fluid), compartment syndrome and rhabdomyolysis.

First-degree burns affect the epidermis and are equivalent to sunburn. They heal without scarring. Partial thickness burns are classified into superficial (affecting the papillary dermis) and deep (affecting the reticular dermis). Superficial partial thickness burns are pink, painful and blanch. They are generally wet and hypersensitive even to air current. They form blisters but do not scar and take around 2 weeks to heal. Deep partial thickness burns are painless and insensate, and do not blanch. They have fixed staining due to capillary thrombosis and take 4–6 weeks to heal because there is a smaller concentration of pilosebaceous glands from which epidermal cells originate.

Tetanus prophylaxis should be considered in all burns patients. Superficial and deep thickness partial burns are treated with agents that chemically debride non-viable tissue, have antibacterial properties and moisture the tissue. The wound should be kept clean and undergo regular review by specialist nurses and plastic surgeons. Full thickness burns can appear white or black and are painless. They affect layers deeper than the dermis and require debridement and superficial thickness skin grafting (autograft down to the dermal layer). Generally, burns patients are not given prophylactic systemic antibiotics but benefit more from topical antibiotics, as eschar that contains bacteria is avascular. Other complications to look out for in burns patients include pneumonia, electrolyte (hyperkalaemia) disturbances, acute kidney injury and acute stress gastric ulcers (Curling's ulcer).

Burns management begins with airway assessment and definitive securement. Look for signs of smoke inhalation such as oropharyngeal oedema or carbon deposits, voice changes, singeing of the eyebrows or nasal hairs as well as obvious burns to the face, neck and chest. Bronchoscopy is the gold standard diagnostic method to evaluate the effect of smoke inhalation on the lungs. Respiratory failure can occur from physical airway obstruction due to pharyngeal oedema and carbon monoxide poisoning, which may manifest as nausea, headache or confusion. If there is no spinal injury, keep the patient elevated at 30 degrees to reduce head and neck oedema. All patients with burns should be administered with 15 L/min of oxygen through a non-rebreather mask with consideration of early orotracheal intubation. High concentration oxygen speeds up the dissociation of carbon monoxide with haemoglobin. Usually, the carbon monoxide–haemoglobin (carboxyhaemoglobin, HbCO) compound's half-life is around 4 hours on room air, but this is reduced to less than 1 hour with supplementary high concentration oxygen. A carboxyhaemoglobin level >60% is associated with very high mortality rates. Obtain baseline arterial blood gas (ABG) analysis and carboxyhaemoglobin levels; do not be reassured by a normal P_aO_2 on an ABG as this is not an accurate predictor of carbon monoxide poisoning. A baseline chest radiograph is also important to track changes in pulmonary function with time. If there are circumferential burns to the chest that restrict the chest wall movement, an emergency chest wall escharotomy may be indicated.

Burn severity is based on the depth of the burn and the total body surface area (BSA). In adults, the BSA can be estimated using the 'rule of nines' or by using the palmar surface including the fingers of a patient's hand to represent approximately 1% of the BSA. Knowing this is important when it comes to fluid resuscitation.

The initial fluid resuscitation for burns patients is extremely important to counter hypovo-laemic shock. It is permissible to place an intravenous cannula through burnt skin, and this is often necessary in extensive injuries. Formulas differ between centres, but the Brooke and Parkland formulae are the commonest. The Brooke formula uses 2 mL and the Parkland formula 4 mL in the equation below:

$$\textit{total fluid in 24 hours} = 2 - 4\,\textit{mL} \times \textit{weight (kg)} \times \textit{total burn surface area (\%)}$$

Half of the fluid is given in the first 8 hours from the time of the injury (not the time of pre-sentation to the ED) and the other half over the remaining 16 hours. The choice of fluid is generally Hartmann's solution. For example, a 70 kg man with 30% total BSA burns requires (2 to 4) × 70 × 30 = 4200 – 8400 mL of Hartmann's over 24 hours. The patient's hourly urinary output should be kept above 0.5 mL/kg/hour for adults, with fluid rate adjusted accordingly. Blood pressure and pulse readings are sometimes difficult to record due to the burns, so urine output becomes an accurate measure of response to fluid resuscitation. There should be a low threshold for considering myoglobinuria or rhabdomyolysis, which also requires aggressive fluid resuscitation and/or sodium bicarbonate infusion.

Alkali burns are more harmful than acidic. They have a longer lasting effect because the body cannot buffer alkali. Electrical burns cause more destruction than the external burn may suggest. They are associated with internal destruction, as the path of least resistance is nerves and blood vessels. They can also cause arrhythmias and an electrocardiogram should be performed.

 Key Points

- Early high concentration oxygen administration helps to prevent and treat hypoxia and carbon monoxide poisoning.
- Early definitive management of the patient's airway (with orotracheal intubation if necessary) is crucial if there are signs of burns in the nose, oropharynx, face or neck. Airway compromise can rapidly develop in these patients.
- Aggressive fluid resuscitation helps to prevent and treat hypovolaemic shock and rhabdomyolysis.

History

An 18-year-old woman attends the Emergency Department with her mother with a history of painful ulcers in her mouth and skin peeling. She reports it starting as a small lip ulcer, but has progressed rapidly and has become increasingly painful, especially when eating or drinking. She has recently returned from holiday and spent a lot of time sun bathing and partying. However, in the past few days, she reports having a fever at times, sore throat and muscle ache. She denies any unprotected sexual intercourse or illicit drug use. She suffers from epilepsy for which she used to use sodium valproate; however, it was recently changed to lamotrigine. She has no allergies and admits to binge drinking during her holiday.

Examination

Vital signs: temperature of 36.6°C, blood pressure of 112/58, heart rate of 105 and regular, respiratory rate of 20, 98% oxygen saturations on air.

The patient has a fair skin type. There are widespread red papules that appear to have erupted on the face and chest. You also note marked blistering and ulcers on the lips and gums.

Questions

1. What is the likely diagnosis?
2. How would you classify the severity of this patient's condition?
3. What are the possible triggers for this condition?
4. What are the complications of this condition?

DISCUSSION

Steven Johnson syndrome (SJS) and toxic epidermal necrolysis (TEN) are considered to be part of a continuous spectrum of a life-threatening mucocutaneous reaction. SJS is defined as epidermal loss of <10% of total body surface area, where as >30% epidermal loss is characterised as severe TEN syndrome, with an overlap syndrome between 10% and 30%. SJS/TEN is rare in the United Kingdom, with an estimated incidence of around 1–2 cases per million with an increased incidence in HLA-B75 positive patients.

Differentials include other bullous and infective disorders such as erythema multiforme, pemphigus vulgaris, pemphigoid syndromes, IgA bullous dermatosis, Staphyloccal scalded skin syndrome (SSSS) and necrotising fasciitis.

SJS/TEN is an acute, potentially life-threatening mucocutaneous disorder characterised by progressive dermal loss and inflammation of mucosal surface. When left untreated, it can result in multi-organ failure. SJS is associated with mortality <10% that rises to 30% for TEN. Patients with SJS/TEN may report prodromal symptoms such as fever, headache, sore throat, malaise and myalgia prior to start of a mucocutaneous eruption. Cutaneous related sensitivity and pain are a particular symptom reported early in the condition. The lesions are variable in appearance and can present from purpuric to 'target' like, occurring on the face, upper torso and proximal aspects of limbs. The lesions may become confluent and begin to shed with minimal shearing force – a positive Nikolsky sign. The shearing of the epidermis exposes the underlying dermis, which oozes serum thereby increasing the risk of secondary infection.

Mucous sites to be aware of include the mouth, eyes and genital areas, which are affected in 90%, 80% and 60% of the cases, respectively. This can result in visual loss, nutritional difficulty and impaired urination and reproductive function in the long term. Other complications include oesophageal strictures, disseminated intravascular coagulation, respiratory failure and acute kidney injury.

The severity of SJS/TEN episode can be assessed with the SCORTEN tool. The following are independent risk factors for death, which each score one point. Five or more points are considered to have a rate of mortality of >90%.

- Age >40 years
- Associated malignancy
- Heart rate >120
- Urea >10 mmol/L
- Initial >10% epidermal loss
- Serum bicarbonate <20 mmol/L
- Serum glucose >14 mmol/L

Immediate management should focus on managing the causative agent (Table 12.1). Blood investigations should include full blood count, ESR, C-reactive protein, renal function, electrolytes (including magnesium, phosphate and bicarbonate), glucose, liver function test, coagulation study and mycoplasma serology should be done. Clinical photography is useful in monitoring mucocutaneous involvement.

Initially manage the large fluid loss from epidermal loss with intravenous fluid resuscitation. Analgesia should be given and titrated as per individual needs. Patient with severe eating difficulties due to oral involvement should have nasogastric tube inserted and feeding

Table 12.1 Common causes for SJS/TEN

Drugs	Infection	Other
Carbamazepine	Viral	Haematological malignancy
Lamotrigine	• Herpes simplex virus (HSV)	Autoimmune disorders
Phenytoin	• Adenovirus	Physical injury or tattoos,
Allopurinol	• Coxsackie	radiotherapy
Sulphur-containing	• Epstein Barr virus (EBV)	Idiopathic
antibiotics	• Cytomegalovirus (CMV)	
Sulphasalazine	Bacterial	
NSAIDS	• Mycoplasma	
	• Streptoccocus	
	• Proteus	
	Fungal	
	• Histoplasmosis	

initiated. Similarly, consider early catheterisation in urological involvement and it will aid in fluid balance monitoring.

Wounds are often difficult to manage without general anaesthesia or potent analgesia such as opioids or ketamine. However, regular warm saline irrigation can be performed with greasy emollient cover and topical antibiotics (as per local guidelines).

Patients with SJS/TEN should be referred to intensive or high dependency care units for specialist nursing. Intensive monitoring and management is required to manage further acute complications and multi-organ failure.

> **Key Points**
>
> - SJS/TEN is rare but life-threatening, analogous to burn injury.
> - Early supportive therapy with fluid and wound management is important for best outcomes.
> - SCORETEN should be calculated on all patients to predict mortality.
> - Multidisciplinary management is required due to multi-system involvement and the wide range of complications – dermatology, critical care, dietician, pharmacist, specialist nurses, ophthalmology and urology.

History

A 19-year-old man has been brought into the Emergency Department as a 'cardiac arrest call'. He appeared to be heavily intoxicated and was seen to be wandering along the canal path late in the evening. Passers-by saw him floating in the water and rescued him. It is thought he was submerged for around 10 minutes in very cold water. There were no signs of life on scene and bystander CPR was started. He has been brought into the ED by a full paramedic crew in cardiac arrest with ongoing CPR. The paramedic crew tell you they have not performed DC cardioversion or given any drugs. Total downtime is now 25 minutes.

Examination

During a pulse check, assessment is as follows:

- A: The patient has a supraglottic airway device inserted and is being ventilated.
- B: There are coarse crackles throughout both lung fields and saturations are unrecordable on high flow oxygen.
- C: There is no palpable pulse and the patient is in asystole. There is an intra-osseous needle inserted into the left proximal humerus.
- D: The GCS is 3/15 and both pupils are fixed at 5 mm.
- E: Core temperature is 29°C and there are no external signs of injury.

Investigations
• Arterial blood gas: pH 7.015, pO_2 35, pCO_2 13, HCO_3 16, BE-10, lactate 9.6, glucose 17.

Questions

1. How are you going to manage this patient?
2. What are the recommendations for DC cardioversion and administration of drugs?
3. When should you consider stopping CPR?

DISCUSSION

This man has suffered a submersion injury and should be managed along Advanced Life Support (ALS) guidelines.

CPR should be continued whilst the paramedics hand the patient over to the receiving ED team, and at the end of the 2-minute CPR cycle, a brief initial assessment should be performed when directed by the team leader. This should be completed in less than 10 seconds and CPR resumed if there is no palpable pulse or signs of life. Ventilation may be carried out via several methods. The simplest is via a bag-valve-mask connected to high flow oxygen. If there are trained practitioners, this should be changed to either a supraglottic device (i-gel®, LMA) or preferably endotracheal intubation as soon as possible. In cases of submersion, this is advantageous as it allows increased positive end expiratory pressure (PEEP), which will recruit collapsed or flooded alveoli. Once this has been established, it is recommended to switch to continuous chest compressions at 100 per minute and ventilation at a rate of 10–12 breaths per minute. There is often concern for concurrent cervical spine injury in these cases, and it may add a layer of complexity into management. Without evidence of diving or head injury, the incidence is around 0.5%, and spinal precautions are not required in every case.

During the resuscitation attempt potentially reversible causes of cardiac arrest should be sought and corrected. They are hypoxia, hypothermia, hypovolaemia, hypo- or hyperkalaemia (and other electrolytes), tension pneumothorax, tamponade, toxins and thromboembolism (4Hs and 4Ts).

This patient is complex and has several potential reversible causes. The submersion injury will almost certainly cause pulmonary oedema by flooding the lungs with contaminated water and mixing with surfactant. Endotracheal intubation and warmed high flow oxygen are keys to reversing hypoxia here.

The alcohol ingestion combined with the prolonged submersion means that the patient may be hypovolaemic. Warmed 0.9% saline or other cystalloid solution should be used to resuscitate the patient. Arterial or venous blood gas testing should be performed as soon as practically possible as it will help to identify any correctible electrolyte disturbances. Heavy alcohol consumption will contribute to a metabolic acidosis as well as cellular hypoxia from the cardiac arrest but should improve with fluid administration. Sodium bicarbonate (8.4%) may be considered for extreme metabolic acidosis in those that fail to improve with fluid resuscitation.

The core temperature was noted to be 29°C, and efforts should be made to rewarm the patient in the ED. Possible options include warmed intravenous fluids, removal of cold wet clothes and forced warm air induction (Baire® hugger). Advanced warming techniques such as bladder lavage, peritoneal lavage or ECMO may be employed if available.

Arrhythmias due to the sudden temperature change may be a contributing cause and if present should be managed per ALS guidelines. Below 30°C, up to three attempts should be made for DC cardioversion and drugs (adrenaline, amiodarone) withheld until core temperature is >30°C. The interval between drug doses should be doubled until core temperature is >34°C.

How long should you continue? There are no fixed criteria but current guidelines suggest that many factors should be considered – the age of the patient, submersion time, temperature of the water and co-morbidities. Younger patients submerged in very cold water (<10°C) may recover with prolonged CPR sometimes longer than 1 hour.

The mantra in the ED is that 'you are not dead until you are warm and dead', and efforts should be made to raise the core temperature to >34°C before making final decisions. Mechanical chest compression devices (e.g. LUCAS®, AutoPulse®) should be considered where prolonged CPR is anticipated as they prevent team fatigue and ideally should be deployed on arrival to the ED.

 Key Points

- The incidence of cervical spine injury in submersion cases is low.
- The team should be prepared for prolonged CPR.
- Drug doses and DC cardioversion thresholds are altered according to core temperature.
- The patient should be warmed to 34°C and all reversible causes corrected before consideration of cessation of CPR.

CASE 14: CRUSHING CENTRAL CHEST PAIN

History

A 62-year-old man is brought to the Emergency Department as a 'priority call' after he developed chest pain. One hour ago, while he was doing some gardening, he started to experience sudden onset, severe central chest pain that did not radiate anywhere. He had associated nausea and sweating, but did not vomit. He has never experienced similar pain in the past. His medical history is notable for type 2 diabetes and hypertension, and there is no family history of cardiac disease. He is a current smoker, but denies any drug use.

Examination

Vital signs: temperature of 36.5°C, heart rate of 75 and regular, blood pressure of 100/60, respiratory rate of 20, 94% O_2 saturation on air.

Physical examination reveals a diaphoretic individual in moderate pain. Radial pulses are equal bilaterally, and cardiorespiratory and abdominal are unremarkable. JVP is not elevated and he has no evidence of peripheral oedema.

🔍 | **Investigations**

- An electrocardiogram (ECG) is shown below.

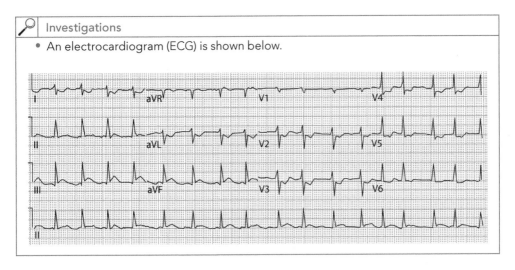

Questions

1. What does the ECG show, and what is the diagnosis?
2. What are the next steps in management that must be performed in the Emergency Department?
3. Would management change if he had presented 3 hours after development of symptoms?

DISCUSSION

This patient has significant cardiac risk factors (smoking, diabetes and hypertension) and presents with acute cardiac-sounding chest pain. Based on the presentation, the treating physician must consider myocardial ischaemia or infarction as the most important diagnosis to exclude, and a 12-lead ECG must be obtained *immediately* in all such patients. Often, the paramedics will have performed a 12 lead ECG, and this must be interpreted if available.

In this case, the ECG shows ST elevation in the inferior leads (II, III and F) as well as reciprocal ST depression in the anterior and lateral leads. This finding, together with the history, is concerning for an ST-elevation myocardial infarction (STEMI), which is a medical emergency. The finding of ECG changes in leads II, III and aVF points towards inferior or posterior wall ischaemia/infarction.

The initial steps to managing this patient should proceed along the 'ABCDE' approach. Supplemental oxygen was traditionally provided even to non-hypoxic patients, but recent evidence suggests it does not provide any benefit and may even harm such individuals. Given the presence of hypotension and possible right ventricular involvement and the absence of signs to suggest pulmonary oedema, an intravenous fluid bolus (250–500 mL) should be administered. Concomitantly, basic blood tests including a full blood count, electrolytes, coagulation screen and troponin must be performed. A chest radiograph is also useful to look for pulmonary oedema, estimate the heart size and exclude thoracic dissection. Pain should be controlled, with morphine being preferred due to its potency and rapid onset of action, and nitrate should also be used, dependent on blood pressure.

The most important goal of the acute management of STEMI is coronary reperfusion, which may be achieved either by percutaneous coronary intervention (PCI) or use of fibrinolytic agents (thrombolysis). PCI is the preferred strategy if it can be delivered within 120 minutes of first medical contact (and ideally within 90 minutes), and would be the best option in this individual. Hospitals may have a STEMI alert/paging system to enable deployment of the primary PCI team, and this should be activated. Prior to PCI, antiplatelet therapy should be administered with a loading dose of aspirin (300 mg) as well as a second anti-platelet agent (e.g. ticagrelor 180 mg or clopidogrel 300 mg).

If there is a delay in presentation to the Emergency Department (e.g. 3 hours after symptom onset), PCI is still the preferred option providing it can be delivered within 120 minutes of *first patient contact* (i.e. door to balloon time). Only if there is an anticipated delay in provision of PCI of >2 hours from first patient contact (e.g. if the patient initially presents to a district hospital without primary PCI capabilities and requires transfer to another centre, with an expected travel time >2 hours) should fibrinolysis be chosen as the reperfusion strategy. This is because several randomised trials have shown that PCI provides improved short- and long-term survival outcomes compared to fibrinolysis, providing it can be performed within the appropriate time frame.

> **🔑 Key Points**
>
> - >1 mm ST elevation in anatomically contiguous lead locations should raise suspicion for ST-elevation myocardial infarction (STEMI).
> - Any patient with a suspected STEMI should be considered for emergent coronary reperfusion via percutaneous coronary intervention (PCI).
> - Prior to PCI, dual anti-platelet therapy, with aspirin 300 mg and either clopidogrel 300 mg or ticagrelor 180 mg, should be administered.
> - The alternative to PCI is thrombolysis, but PCI is preferred providing it can be performed within 120 minutes of first patient contact.

INTERNAL MEDICINE

CASE 15: SHORT OF BREATH AND TIGHT IN THE CHEST

History

A 20-year-old woman is brought in as a 'priority call' to the Emergency Department. She has become increasingly short of breath over the last few hours and complains of a 'tight' feeling in her chest. She has a history of asthma managed with regular use of inhaled beclomethasone and salbutamol as needed. Today, she has used her salbutamol inhaler on multiple occasions, but it has provided minimal relief. She has never previously been admitted to hospital with an asthma attack and has no other medical comorbidities.

Examination

Vital signs: temperature of 36.0°C, blood pressure of 110/60, heart rate of 120 and regular, respiratory rate of 25, 94% O_2 saturations on air.

Physical examination reveals an anxious-appearing slim female who has difficulty completing sentences in one full breath. Respiratory examination is notable for widespread expiratory wheeze.

 Investigations

- An arterial blood gas performed on arrival (with the patient breathing room air) shows pH 7.43, pO_2 8.2, pCO_2 4.0, HCO_3 22.
- Peak expiratory flow rate is 200 L/min (predicted 450 L/min).

Questions

1. What is the diagnosis, and how would you classify the severity of this patient's condition?
2. Outline the next steps in managing this patient. How would you monitor treatment response?
3. Would your management change if the initial ABG (on room air) showed pH 7.45, pO_2 7.8, pCO_2 4.8, HCO_3 22?
4. Is there any role for assisted ventilation in this patient?

DISCUSSIONS

The history and examination findings in this patient are suggestive of an acute exacerbation of asthma. Asthma is a condition characterised by airway obstruction due to bronchial smooth muscle constriction and inflammation that is at least partly reversible. Any asthmatic is susceptible to suffering from an exacerbation ('asthma attack'), which may be caused by allergic triggers (e.g. pollen, mould), respiratory infection, medications (e.g. NSAIDs or β-blockers) or lack of compliance with treatment.

The severity of an asthma exacerbation is based upon objective parameters and should always be evaluated in any asthmatic presenting to the ED. A moderate asthma exacerbation describes asthmatics with increased symptoms and a peak expiratory flow rate (PEFR) of >50% than their best or predicted value. Acute severe asthma describes an individual with *any* of the following features:

    a. PEFR 33%–50% best or predicted value
    b. Respiratory rate ≥25/min
    c. Heart rate ≥110/min
    d. Inability to complete sentences in one full breath

Our patient meets all four criteria and should be considered as a case of acute severe asthma.

Initial management of a patient with acute severe asthma should follow the 'ABCDE' algorithm and comprises of three key interventions:

    i. Oxygen. Supplemental oxygen should be administered, with titration of flow rate to maintain O_2 saturations between 94% and 98%.
    ii. Nebulisers. Bronchodilators, namely β_2-agonists such as salbutamol, should be given, preferably with an oxygen-driven nebulising device, with the aim of relieving bronchoconstriction. Bolus nebulisation with 2.5–5 mg salbutamol usually achieves good response in most exacerbations, though repeated boluses or addition of an anticholinergic (0.5 mg ipratropium, in the form of 'back-to-back nebs') may be needed if response to initial therapy is poor.
    iii. Steroids. The aim is to reduce airway inflammation, though it must be noted that their onset of action will be in the order of a few hours. Intravenous hydrocortisone (e.g. 100 mg every 6 hours) would be appropriate for acute severe asthma, whereas oral prednisolone (40 mg daily) would suffice for a moderate exacerbation.

Arguably the most important aspect of managing acute severe asthma is monitoring response to interventions. Regular measurements of PEFR and blood gases, together with clinical assessment (symptoms, degree of wheeze, ability to complete sentences, oxygen saturations), are required to ensure that patients who are not responding adequately are identified promptly. In situations where there is a poor response to initial therapy, there is limited evidence for adjunctive therapies such as intravenous magnesium or aminophylline, and these should only be used after consulting with senior physicians.

It is essential that treating physicians are able to identify life-threatening asthma, which includes *any* of the following features:

    a. Clinical – altered consciousness, signs of exhaustion, poor respiratory effort, hypotension, cyanosis, silent chest or evidence of arrhythmia

b. Objective parameters – PEFR <33% predicted, O_2 saturations <92%, pO_2 <8 kPa or a 'normal' pCO_2 (4.5–6 kPa, indicating respiratory fatigue with inability to maintain hyperventilation as a mechanism to boost oxygenation)

Asthma is fundamentally an airway pathology, and therefore, evidence of any of the above (or even where an asthmatic has not responded well to initial therapy but does not yet meet criteria for life-threatening disease) should prompt early and urgent referral to Intensive Care. Assisted ventilation may be required in up to 5% of patients with severe asthma; the majority of these individuals require intubation and mechanical ventilation, although non-invasive positive pressure ventilation (NIV) has also been shown to have some beneficial impact. Even when patients are intubated or receiving NIV, it is important to continue nebulised bronchodilators and steroids as these are the disease-modifying therapies – the purpose of mechanical ventilation is to maintain adequate oxygenation and reduce work of breathing whilst waiting for these therapies to exert their effects. Despite these efforts, the prognosis for asthmatics admitted to the Intensive Care Unit is guarded, with an in-hospital mortality of 7% in those who are mechanically ventilated. It is therefore vital that clinicians managing asthma in the ED are wary of the potential for deterioration and have no hesitation in involving senior physicians and/or the Intensive Care team if initial therapy does not appear to be effective.

 Key Points

- Asthma exacerbations are a common presentation to the Emergency Department, and initial assessment must include measurement of the PEFR, with comparison to a patient's best or predicted value.
- Oxygen, nebulised bronchodilators and intravenous or oral steroids are the key steps in managing acute severe asthma.
- A tiring asthmatic with an inappropriately normal or rising pCO_2 indicates life-threatening disease, and urgent referral to the Intensive Care Unit for potential mechanical ventilation is required.

CASE 16: A PRODUCTIVE COUGH

History

A 71-year-old man is brought to the Emergency Department as a 'priority call' with a 3-day history of shortness of breath. He reports a cough that has become increasingly productive of green-coloured sputum, which is different to what he normally brings up. He has a history of moderate COPD and has been using his home nebulisers regularly for the past few days, but to little effect.

Examination

Vital signs: temperature of 37.5°C, blood pressure of 110/70, heart rate of 120 and regular, respiratory rate of 32, 87% O_2 saturation on room air.

Physical examination reveals a slim man, who is markedly dyspnoeic at rest. Cardiopulmonary examination is notable for widespread polyphonic wheeze.

 Investigations

- An arterial blood gas (ABG) on air reveals pH 7.28, pO_2 6.9, pCO_2 6.7, HCO_3 28.

Questions

1. What is the likely diagnosis, and what investigations would you perform in the ED?
2. Describe the results of the ABG, and outline the initial management of this patient.
3. After 1 hour, a repeat ABG shows pH 7.29, pO_2 7.3, pCO_2 6.5, HCO_3 28. What would you consider next, and what factors need to be taken into account at this point?

DISCUSSION

This patient is experiencing an acute exacerbation of COPD, most probably triggered by an infection. COPD is a disorder characterised by *irreversible* airflow obstruction, and patients are vulnerable to suffering exacerbations, clinical features of which include worsening dyspnoea and cough, and a change in sputum production or colour. The latter generally indicate an infective cause and are likely in this patient, with common pathogens being bacterial (notably *Haemophilus influenzae, Streptococcus pneumoniae, Moraxella catarrhalis*) and viral (influenza, rhinovirus, respiratory syncytial virus). When an (infective) exacerbation is suspected, important investigations to perform at first presentation include a full blood count, electrolytes and liver function, arterial blood gas (ABG), blood cultures (particularly if the patient is febrile), sputum cultures, an electrocardiogram and a chest radiograph. Of these, an ABG is particularly important to assess for respiratory failure, and it is important to compare with prior ABGs to see if there has been a change from baseline.

Acute management of a COPD exacerbation should follow the 'ABCDE' algorithm. Supplemental oxygen should be provided in a controlled manner, with the aim of keeping O_2 saturations between 88% and 92%. In this case, the initial ABG shows an acidotic type 2 respiratory failure (hypoxaemia with hypercapnia), with an elevated HCO_3 suggesting chronic metabolic compensation; hence, it is important not to over-oxygenate the patient to avoid removing the hypoxic central respiratory stimulus. Short-acting bronchodilators administered via nebuliser (e.g. 2.5 mg salbutamol and 500 µg ipratropium) should be used to try and open up smaller airways, whilst systemic corticosteroids (typically 30 mg oral prednisolone) should be commenced to reduce airway inflammation. It is common to use a short course (5–7 days) of steroids, although it may be necessary to taper off gently if the patient was using these prior to presentation. Finally, in this patient, antibiotics should be commenced given the likelihood of an infective exacerbation; antibiotic choice is guided by local policies but normally comprises of a penicillin and macrolide (for atypical coverage) or doxycycline. Ideally, all these interventions should be initiated within the first hour of presentation, with repeat assessment including blood gases performed afterwards.

In this case, despite optimal medical management, type 2 respiratory failure with acidosis persists and the patient may meet indications for non-invasive ventilation (NIV) in the form of bi-level positive airway pressure (BiPAP) support. The indication for NIV is ongoing respiratory acidosis (pH 7.26–7.35 with pCO_2 >6 kPa) despite maximal standard medical therapy for 1 hour or more. NIV reduces respiratory rate and the work of breathing, and can therefore improve respiratory acidosis and reduce the need for invasive ventilation.

Before deciding on trialing NIV, it is important to set ceilings of care by assessing the patient's pre-morbid and current state, the reversibility of the current condition, the presence of any contraindications to NIV and also the patient's wishes or advance care directives. A decision to undertake NIV should not be taken lightly, and clinicians should always ask themselves if the patient is a candidate for intubation, and if care should be ward- or ICU-based. Indeed, in some circumstances, it may be appropriate to pursue full medical management without NIV or even to elect for palliative care in highly comorbid patients with severe disease.

Important inclusion criteria for NIV include the ability of patients to protect their own airway and to be conscious and co-operative, as well as there being the potential to recover a quality of life acceptable to the patient. Contraindications to NIV include any facial burns or trauma, fixed upper airway obstruction, pneumothorax, inability to protect the airway, copious respiratory secretions, severe comorbidity and haemodynamic instability requiring inotropes or vasopressors unless the patient is being managed in an intensive care setting.

Once a decision has been made to commence NIV, initial settings often use an inspiratory positive airway pressure (IPAP) of 10–12 cm H_2O with an expiratory positive airway pressure (EPAP) of 4–6 cm H_2O, which are well tolerated by most patients. It is common to up-titrate the IPAP in increments of 2–3 cm H_2O until the limit of patient tolerability is reached. It is also important to remember that oxygen can continue to be delivered to the patient whilst administering NIV, and should be appropriately titrated to maintain saturations between 88% and 92%. A repeat ABG within 1 hour of NIV initiation is required to assess response and help guide further changes in NIV settings or even goals of care, and should always be performed 1 hour after any change in settings.

Key Points

- COPD exacerbations are common and characterised by worsening shortness of breath and a change in sputum volume and/or colour.
- Medical management for exacerbations comprises controlled oxygen therapy (to maintain saturations between 88% and 92%), nebulised bronchodilators and steroids. Antibiotics should be given if an infective cause is suspected.
- NIV should be considered in suitable patients with persisting respiratory acidosis despite optimum medical management, and ceilings of care should be assessed prior to its commencement.

CASE 17: A COLLAPSE AT WORK

History

A 60-year-old man is brought in to the Emergency Department after collapsing at work. His colleagues report that he complained of feeling short of breath just before he collapsed. He has a history of multiple myeloma and is on oral maintenance chemotherapy. He is a smoker, but has no pertinent family history of note.

Examination

Vital signs: temperature of 37.2°C, blood pressure of 85/50, heart rate of 110 and regular, respiratory rate of 28, 94% O_2 saturation on 6 L/min.

The patient is conscious, with a GCS of 15. The extremities are cool, capillary refill time is 2 s and cardiorespiratory examination is unremarkable apart from an elevated JVP. The left leg is mildly swollen but is not tender to touch.

 Investigations

- ABG (on 6 L/min): pH 7.47, pO_2 8.5, pCO_2 3.7, HCO_3 24.
- An electrocardiogram (ECG) shows sinus tachycardia with right bundle branch block, which appears new compared to prior ECGs. A portable chest radiograph shows no focal consolidation.

Questions

1. What is the differential diagnosis, and based on the clinical information, what is the most likely diagnosis?
2. Describe the initial approach to managing this patient in the Emergency Department.
3. What treatment should be considered, and are further investigations needed before pursuing this?

DISCUSSION

This patient presents with shortness of breath and a syncopal episode (i.e. collapse). The key diagnoses to consider are cardiopulmonary, including acute coronary syndromes (ACS), pulmonary embolism (PE), cardiac disease (e.g. aortic stenosis, hypertrophic cardiomyopathy, dissection), as well as more benign conditions such as a vasovagal episode. In this case, the most likely diagnosis is a massive pulmonary embolism, based on the history (active malignancy, current smoker), examination findings (signs suggestive of left leg deep venous thrombosis and poor oxygenation) and investigations (sinus tachycardia, new right bundle branch block, hypoxaemia).

The initial approach to managing this patient should proceed along the 'ABCDE' approach. Here, given that the patient is hypoxaemic, additional O_2 should be delivered by a non-rebreathe mask, and intravenous access secured to enable administration of a fluid bolus. Baseline blood tests including a full blood count, electrolytes, clotting screen (d-dimer may be elevated due to myeloma) and group and save should be performed. As the patient is profoundly hypoxic and hypotensive, an early referral to intensive care should be made.

The definitive investigation to diagnose PE is CT pulmonary angiography (CTPA), but in this case, there is evidence of haemodynamic instability and circulatory collapse. It would therefore be unsafe to pursue a CTPA in this patient, unless there is evidence of haemodynamic improvement after fluid resuscitation. In such an instance, a point of care echocardiogram to assess for right ventricular strain or possibly to visualise the thrombus may be useful to help confirm the diagnosis, but only if performed by a trained and experienced practitioner.

In patients with suspected massive PE who are haemodynamically *unstable* or shocked as in our case, thrombolytic therapy with intravenous alteplase 10 mg followed by an infusion of 90 mg over 2 hours is indicated. Ideally, it should only be used once the diagnosis of PE is confirmed, but this may not always be feasible. Other, less strong, indications for thrombolysis in PE include haemodynamically *stable* patients with severe right ventricular dysfunction, extensive clot burden and cardiopulmonary arrest due to PE. It is also important to be aware of contraindications to thrombolysis, which include intracranial neoplasm, history of a haemorrhagic stroke and active bleeding diathesis. If thrombolysis is unsuccessful (i.e. the patient continues to be haemodynamically unstable), consideration could be given towards catheter-directed thrombolytic therapy or surgical embolectomy.

 Key Points

- Obstructive cardiopulmonary disease is the main diagnosis to exclude in patients presenting with shortness of breath and syncope.
- A CTPA is performed to confirm a diagnosis of pulmonary embolism (PE), but should only be done when the patient is haemodynamically stable.
- Thrombolysis is indicated in haemodynamically unstable patients with evidence of a massive PE, but beware of contraindications such as history of a brain tumour or haemorrhagic stroke.

History

A 70-year-old woman is referred by her General Practitioner to the Emergency Department with a 3-day history of dysuria and urinary frequency. At the GP visit, she reported feeling weak and was found to be febrile, prompting evaluation in secondary care. She has a history of type 2 diabetes, managed with metformin, and suffers from frequent urinary tract infections. She lives in a residential care home with her husband.

Examination

Vital signs: temperature of 38.5°C, blood pressure of 80/40, heart rate of 110 and regular, respiratory rate of 20, 95% O_2 saturations on air.

Physical examination reveals an ill-looking woman who is somnolent. The extremities are cool, capillary refill time is 2 seconds and cardiac and respiratory examinations are unremarkable. Abdominal examination is notable for suprapubic tenderness. There are no focal neurologic signs, but the abbreviated mental test (AMT) score is 5/10.

Questions

1. What are the diagnosis and the likely underlying cause?
2. What are the next steps in investigating and managing this patient?
3. What factors can help predict the risk of poor outcomes in this patient?

DISCUSSION

This patient exhibits several of the cardinal symptoms and signs of sepsis. This is a syndrome arising from a dysregulated inflammatory response to infection in this case, most likely a urinary tract infection and which has the potential to lead to organ dysfunction. Historically, systemic inflammatory response syndrome (SIRS) criteria were used in defining sepsis and its severity, but these have been excluded from latest consensus guidelines as SIRS is not always caused by infection. The main clinical features of sepsis include hypotension (systolic blood pressure <80 mm Hg), tachycardia (pulse >90), a high (>38.3°C) or low (<36°C) temperature, altered mental status and signs of peripheral shutdown (cool skin, prolonged capillary refill, cyanosis) in severe cases.

Sepsis is an extremely important condition to recognise as it is associated with high morbidity and mortality (up to 50%). Prompt recognition and intervention is therefore required. The 'Surviving Sepsis' campaign recommends that the following six interventions (so-called 'Sepsis Six') be performed within the *first hour* of a patient suspected to be septic, and which have been shown to improve mortality outcomes:

    i. Delivering of high-flow oxygen
    ii. Obtaining blood cultures
    iii. Measurement of lactate
    iv. Commencing intravenous fluid resuscitation
    v. Administration of broad-spectrum antibiotics
    vi. Obtaining accurate measurement of urine output (typically with urethral catheterisation)

These interventions are designed to stabilise respiration with oxygen, look for infectious causes and possibly isolate the causative pathogen with blood cultures and assess organ hypoperfusion with the lactate and urine output. Intravenous fluid resuscitation helps restore intravascular volume and should be administered in a 'bolus' fashion (e.g. 500 mL) with sequential fluid challenges and reassessment by means of the blood pressure, heart rate, lactate and clinical status. Randomised trials have shown no difference in outcomes between crystalloid solutions and albumin, but the former is typically used. Central venous access may be required, either due to the need to monitor venous pressures and gauge response to fluid resuscitation more accurately, or due to difficulty in securing peripheral access. Broad-spectrum antibiotics should be used in all septic patients until cultures allow tailoring of the anti-microbial regime, and a regimen such as vancomycin and piperacillin-tazobactam would be appropriate to ensure coverage of Gram positive (including MRSA) and negative organisms, though each hospital may have its own guidelines. Additional investigations that should be performed include checking the full blood count and renal function, cultures of other relevant sites (e.g. urine culture or possibly lumbar puncture if meningitis is suspected) and screening for other sources of infection (e.g. chest radiograph).

Sepsis is associated with substantial in-hospital morbidity and mortality, and an increased risk of death and re-admission to hospital even if the patient survives until discharge. Prognostic factors in sepsis include patient factors (increasing age, higher comorbidity), site of infection (urosepsis is associated with better outcomes compared to other sources), type of pathogen (nosocomial infections have higher mortality), early administration of antibiotics (which may reduce mortality by 50%) and restoration of perfusion. A modified version of the Sequential Organ Failure Assessment (SOFA) score termed quick SOFA, or qSOFA, has also recently been proposed to help identify patients at risk of death, and this relies on three components (respiratory rate ≥22, altered mental status and systolic blood pressure ≤100 mm Hg), with a score of 2 or more associated with poorer outcomes.

 Key Points

- Sepsis is a syndrome caused by a dysregulated inflammatory response to infection and can lead to multi-organ dysfunction and death.
- The 'Sepsis Six' has been shown to improve mortality from sepsis and consists of three diagnostic (measurement of lactate, measurement of urine output, obtaining blood cultures) and three therapeutic (high-flow oxygen, intravenous fluids and broad-spectrum antibiotics) interventions that should be performed within 1 hour of diagnosis.

History

A 55-year-old woman is sent by her General Practitioner to the Emergency Department after presenting with a 3-week history of worsening shortness of breath, swelling in her legs and weight gain of 10 kg. She denies any chest pain and has no history of cardiovascular disease. She also denies any urinary or gastrointestinal symptoms. Family history is significant for rheumatoid arthritis in her two sisters.

Examination

Vital signs: temperature of 36.7°C, blood pressure of 105/70, heart rate of 90 and regular, respiratory rate of 24, 93% O_2 saturation on air.

She is dyspnoeic on talking sentences, but is alert and oriented. Cardiac examination is notable for elevated JVP (+6 cm), and respiratory examination is notable for crackles at both lung bases. Abdominal examination is normal. There is pitting oedema up to both knees.

 Investigations

- Hb 11.4, WCC 8.5, PLT 220, Na 131, K 6.4, Ur 35, Cr 220, HCO_3 18. Venous pH is 7.25. Review of the records show that Cr was 80 when last checked 5 months ago.
- A chest radiograph shows small bilateral pleural effusions and congested lung fields.
- She is admitted to the High Dependency Unit (HDU).

Questions

1. What do you suspect is the diagnosis, and what investigations should be performed next?
2. Outline the initial steps of management in the HDU.
3. Does the patient require renal replacement therapy? Justify your response.

DISCUSSION

This patient presents symptoms and signs of fluid overload and laboratory evaluation notable for evidence of acute kidney injury (AKI), with associated hyponatraemia, hyperkalaemia and metabolic acidosis. There are various definitions of AKI, with the Kidney Disease: Improving Global Outcomes (KDIGO) defining AKI by any one of the following:

   i. Increase in serum creatinine (Cr) by ≥26.5 μmol/L within 48 hours
   ii. Increase in serum Cr to ≥1.5 × baseline, which is known or presumed to have occurred in the preceding 7 days
   iii. Urine output <0.5 mL/kg/hour for 6 hours

In this patient, we know that the baseline Cr was 80 μmol/L and therefore the current value of 220 μmol/L represents an AKI as it is nearly three times the baseline level.

Classically, there are three major causative categories of AKI: (i) pre-renal (i.e. hypoperfusion), (ii) renal (i.e. an intrinsic process with the kidneys) and (iii) post-renal (i.e. urinary tract obstruction). The initial evaluation should attempt to determine which of these are leading to AKI in the patient. Urinalysis is essential and must be performed immediately as it can help identify evidence of an intra-renal process (e.g. presence of red cell casts with glomerulonephritis, white cell casts with interstitial nephritis or renal epithelial cells in the case of acute tubular necrosis). The second key investigation is a renal ultrasound to look for obstruction, which will be manifested by the identification of hydronephrosis and/or hydro-ureter. Based on these, further investigations can then be performed, such as serologic testing for glomerulonephritides.

The initial management of this patient in the HDU should focus on the two main complications that arise with AKI – volume and electrolyte issues. With regard to volume status, a urinary catheter should be inserted to enable accurate measurement of urine output, and there should be hourly documentation of fluid intake, output and balance. This patient clinically appears to be volume overloaded and the chest radiograph also supports this. Therefore, she should be diuresed, both to relieve symptoms but also to see the effect on urine output. Intravenous furosemide is the diuretic of choice, with a dose of 40–80 mg typically used in diuretic-naïve patients, and the dose should be doubled if there is a lack of response.

The electrolyte abnormalities that merit attention in this patient are hyponatraemia (likely due to hypervolaemia), hyperkalaemia and metabolic acidosis. The latter two arise as a result of reduced potassium and acid excretion by the kidneys as a result of tubular damage. Hyponatraemia will resolve with fluid removal (via diuresis), but hyperkalaemia must be promptly treated (with insulin/dextrose, calcium gluconate and possibly a potassium resin). Furosemide will help lower potassium, assuming the patient is still making urine. Acidosis can be treated with administration of bicarbonate, but will resolve as the AKI is treated; in this situation, it may therefore be preferable to pursue evaluation and treatment of the cause of the AKI and monitor acid–base balance rather than proceeding with bicarbonate infusion.

The key indications for renal replacement therapy (RRT) in AKI include (i) fluid overload that is refractory to diuresis, (ii) hyperkalaemia refractory to medical therapy, (iii) metabolic acidosis (pH <7.1) and (iv) complications arising from uraemia (e.g. encephalopathy, pericarditis). This patient may require RRT (in the form of haemodialysis or continuous veno-venous haemofiltration) but should first be treated for volume overload and hyperkalaemia as outlined above. If she does not respond to these interventions (in terms of fluid balance, hyperkalaemia and acidosis) or her clinical condition deteriorates (e.g. development of encephalopathy), RRT would be indicated.

Key Points

- Acute kidney injury (AKI) is commonly seen in patients presenting to the Emergency Department.
- It may be caused by pre-renal, intra-renal or post-renal processes, and a urinalysis and renal ultrasound should be obtained to help differentiate between these.
- Indications for renal replacement therapy in AKI include fluid overload, refractory hyperkalaemia, metabolic acidosis and uraemic complications.

History

A 25-year-old man of African descent presents to the Emergency Department with a 3-day history of worsening right-sided chest pain. He complains of generalised and severe pain in his arms and legs, as well as shortness of breath and a dry cough. He has a history of sickle cell disease and has been maintained on hydroxyurea for the last few years. He denies any recent travel or infectious exposure.

Examination

Vital signs: temperature of 38.0°C, blood pressure of 110/65, heart rate of 95 and regular, respiratory rate of 26, 90% O_2 saturation on air.

General examination reveals an ill-appearing man who is in acute pain. Cardiac examination is normal, but respiratory examination is notable for crackles at the right lower zone.

	Investigations

- Hb 7.2, WCC 15.4 (neutrophils 11.5), PLT 435, Na 143, K 4.2, Ur 9, Cr 90.
- Arterial blood gas (on air): pH 7.40, pO_2 7.7, pCO_2 4.5, HCO_3 23.
- A chest radiograph shows increased opacification in the lower zones of the right lung.

Questions

1. What is the most likely diagnosis?
2. What are the likely causes of this presentation?
3. How should the patient be managed in the Emergency Department? Should he receive a blood transfusion?

DISCUSSION

Vaso-occlusive crises are one of the important complications of sickle cell disease, and arise as a result of sickled red blood cells pooling in blood vessels, leading to vascular obstruction. This patient likely has vaso-occlusion in the pulmonary vessels, and is suffering from acute chest syndrome, a condition that will affect 50% of sickle cell patients in their disease course.

Acute chest syndrome is diagnosed by the presence of radiologic evidence of consolidation, in addition to at least one of the following: fever ≥38.5°C, >2% decrease in O_2 saturations from a steady state on room air, cough, chest pain, wheezing, use of accessory muscles of respiration, tachypnoea, auscultation of crackles and pO_2 <8 kPa. This patient presents with chest pain and cough, and has evidence of tachypnoea and hypoxaemia, as well as unilateral findings on a chest radiograph; he therefore meets the criteria for acute chest syndrome. This may be precipitated by various factors, including infection (often with atypical organisms such as *Mycoplasma*), fat emboli as a result of bone marrow ischaemia and necrosis, and hypoventilation, which may arise due to over-sedation from opioid analgesics or reduced inspiratory effort as a result of bone infarcts in the ribs or sternum.

The acute management of acute chest syndrome initially involves prompt recognition and consideration of this as a diagnosis in patients with sickle cell disease presenting with respiratory symptoms and/or signs. Pain control is a key part of initial treatment and often will require high doses of opiate analgesics. A personalised analgesia protocol for known sickle cell patients may be stored in the ED and/or haematology records and should be consulted if available. Fluid resuscitation is often required as patients may be dehydrated or have super-added chest sepsis; however, it is important to avoid over-hydration as this may precipitate pulmonary oedema. Supplementary oxygen should be provided in all patients with acute chest syndrome who have O_2 saturations <92% or a pO_2 of <9.3 kPa, and aggressive pulmonary hygiene with incentive spirometry and the use of bronchodilators should be initiated. Finally, empiric antibiotics with atypical coverage should be initiated as infection is a common precipitant of acute chest syndrome, and a basic evaluation (e.g. sputum culture, Streptococcal and Legionella urinary antigens) performed to help tailor anti-microbial therapy.

Blood transfusion is one of the key aspects of managing acute chest syndrome, with the aim being to not only increase the oxygen-carrying capacity of the blood but also reduce the percentage of sickled red blood cells (i.e. HbS), thereby reducing the likelihood of further vaso-occlusion. Simple blood transfusion can be used in mild cases, where the goal should be to raise the haemoglobin to around 10 g/dL. Exchange transfusion, where the patient's blood is removed and replaced with donor blood is used in more severe cases (e.g. multi-lobar lung involvement, marked hypoxia, clinical deterioration, lack of response to simple transfusion), with the aim again to raise haemoglobin to a target of 10 g/dL. In this patient, simple transfusion of 2 units of red blood cells would be indicated given uni-lobar involvement and absence of marked hypoxaemia, but he should be carefully monitored for deterioration in which case there should be no delay in performing exchange transfusion.

Severe acute chest syndrome may be complicated by pulmonary infarcts and vaso-occlusive crises (PE), and appropriate imaging should be carried out when this is suspected. Early consultation with haematology is essential, and these patients are managed best in a high dependency setting as they may have cardiac complications (cardiomyopathy, heart failure) associated with sickle cell disease.

> **Key Points**
>
> - Sickle cell patients are vulnerable to having vaso-occlusive episodes leading to severe pain.
> - Acute chest syndrome is a vaso-occlusive episode within the lungs and may be precipitated by infection, fat emboli or hypoventilation.
> - Any patient suspected to have acute chest syndrome should be discussed with haematology to determine whether simple or exchange blood transfusion is needed.

History

A 35-year-old woman presents to the Emergency Department with a 3-day history of feeling generally unwell and weak. She has also noted a new rash on her arms and legs, and felt feverish earlier today. She has no other medical history and does not take any regular medications.

Examination

Vital signs: temperature of 38.5°C, heart rate of 110 and regular, blood pressure of 90/50, respiratory rate of 16, 95% O₂ saturation on air.

Physical examination is notable for a blanching petechial rash on her extremities, conjunctival pallor and cool extremities. The cardiac and respiratory examinations are unremarkable.

 Investigations

- Hb 7.5, MCV 85, WCC 12 (neutrophils 9.5), PLT 10, Na 137, K 4.3, Ur 8.5, Cr 160, bilirubin 40, ALT 35, AST 65, ALP 87.
- A blood film is shown below.
- The patient is admitted to the Intensive Care Unit for further monitoring and treatment.

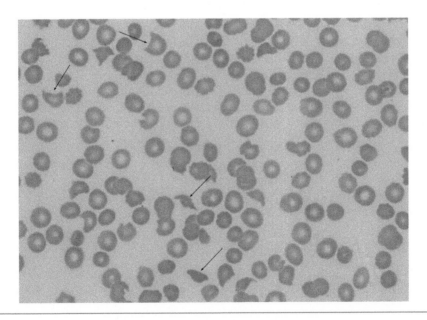

Questions

1. What is the most important diagnosis to consider in this case? What does the blood film show?
2. What investigations should be performed to confirm the diagnosis?
3. How should the patient be treated, and how is response to treatment monitored?

DISCUSSION

This patient presents with relatively non-specific symptoms, including fever, and has evidence of thrombocytopaenia, haemolytic anaemia and renal failure, the constellation of which should alert clinicians to a diagnosis of thrombotic thrombocytopaenic purpura (TTP). TTP is a thrombotic microangiopathy caused by deficiency of the ADAMTS13 protease, an enzyme that cleaves von Willebrand factor (VWF) multimers from endothelial cells. The deficiency of this enzyme leads to development of platelet thrombi in small vessels, producing haemolytic anaemia and thrombocytopaenia. Clinical manifestations such as renal failure are a result of vascular or ischaemic insult to the various organ systems, but it is important to note that the classically described pentad of fever, haemolytic anaemia, thrombocytopaenia, renal failure and neurologic changes is only seen in a small fraction of cases of TTP.

The key investigations that need to be performed include evaluation of the anaemia and thrombocytopaenia by means of a blood film, that shows schistocytes and helmet cells, indicative of red cell fragmentation, and identification of other features of haemolysis by measuring LDH and total bilirubin, both of which will be elevated. It is also important to exclude TTP mimics such as disseminated intravascular coagulation (DIC) by confirming that there is no coagulopathy (PT and APTT should be normal in TTP, but will typically be elevated in DIC). The key diagnostic test for TTP is measurement of ADAMTS13 activity, with a level of <5% indicating severe deficiency and being diagnostic for TTP.

As platelet thrombi may form in any vessel of the body (e.g. brain, heart, kidney), TTP is a medical emergency and treatment should be initiated if there is a strong suspicion of the diagnosis, even whilst awaiting results of confirmatory testing (ADAMTS13 activity). The mainstay of treatment is daily plasma exchange (PLEX), often in combination with glucocorticoids (prednisolone 1 mg/kg). Central access is required for PLEX, which aims to replenish ADAMTS13 and/or remove autoantibodies that are inhibiting its activity, and urgent involvement of haematology and/or nephrology is therefore needed.

Response to treatment is assessed by monitoring the platelet count, with normalisation expected after a week of therapy, at which point PLEX may be discontinued; glucocorticoids are typically tapered off more slowly over a period of 2–3 weeks. However, it is important to monitor the patient closely for any signs of bleeding or thrombosis, particularly during the first few days of therapy, as TTP induces a pro-coagulant state whilst thrombocytopaenia can predispose to spontaneous haemorrhage.

 Key Points

- The presence of thrombocytopaenia and haemolytic anaemia should raise the suspicion for TTP.
- TTP is a medical emergency caused by deficiency of the ADAMTS13 protease, leading to development of platelet thrombi.
- Treatment with plasma exchange and glucocorticoids must be initiated urgently if the diagnosis is suspected, even whilst awaiting the results of confirmatory testing.

History

A 65-year-old man is brought in as a 'priority call' to the Emergency Department after he fainted at home. He was found by his wife on the commode and she told paramedics that his stools were bright red in colour. His wife reports that he had mentioned having blood in his stools over the past couple of days as well. He has a history of atrial fibrillation and has been on warfarin for the past 4 years. He was recently treated by his GP for a chest infection with clarithromycin, and has a history of hypertension and previous myocardial infarction.

Examination

Vital signs: temperature of 36.4°C, blood pressure of 90/55, heart rate of 105 and irregular, respiratory rate of 18, 94% O_2 saturation on air.

General examination reveals an ill-looking man who is not in acute distress. The peripheries are cool and CRT is 2 seconds. Cardiorespiratory examination is unremarkable, and there is mild tenderness in the lower abdomen. Rectal examination is positive for dark red blood with the presence of clots.

Investigations
• Hb 6.7, WCC 8.5, PLT 195, Na 134, K 3.7, Ur 9, Cr 80, INR 5.5.

Questions

1. How would you manage this patient acutely?
2. What are the possible reasons for the elevated INR? Does the INR require correction, and if so, how?
3. Describe how management would change if he had no bleeding and the INR was 5.5. What if there was no bleeding and the INR was elevated but less than 5?

DISCUSSION

This patient presents what appears to be lower gastrointestinal (GI) bleeding, as evidenced by fresh blood in his stools and the presence of clots on rectal examination. He is tachycardic and hypotensive, and also has an elevated INR. He should be acutely managed in the resuscitation room as he is unstable; management should proceed along the 'ABCDE' approach, with delivery of supplemental oxygen and establishment of intravenous access with two large-bore cannulae. A fluid bolus (e.g. 1 L of normal saline) should be administered and blood should be sent for cross-match. Packed red cells (either blood group O or fully cross-matched blood if time allows) may be used also as this patient is clearly shocked and has a history of cardiac disease with the aim to maintain haemoglobin >8 g/dL. There should then be discussion with Gastroenterology and/or Interventional Radiology to consider intervention by means of lower GI endoscopy and/or angiography with embolisation.

One of the key aspects of managing this patient's blood is addressing his coagulopathy (elevated INR). Warfarin is associated with a 1%–3% risk of bleeding each year in patients with atrial fibrillation, and the main risk factors for this include presence of comorbidities, interacting medications, poor patient compliance, acute illness and dietary variation in vitamin K intake. In this patient, the most likely explanation for the elevated INR is concurrent use of clarithromycin, which inhibits hepatic metabolism of warfarin, thereby leading to higher drug levels.

Management of a supratherapeutic INR depends upon two factors: (i) the extent of INR elevation and (ii) the presence or absence of bleeding. In the presence of serious or life-threatening bleeding (as in this patient), complete reversal is required within a short period of time. This is achieved by administration of prothrombin complex concentrate (PCC, e.g. Octaplex®), which contains factors II, VII, IX and X; dosing depends on INR, but is typically between 25 and 50 units/kg. PCC can reverse INR very quickly, but the factors they contain have a short half-life, and therefore, IV vitamin K (5–10 mg) should also be given in this case. It is important to note that fresh frozen plasma (FFP) leads to suboptimal INR reversal as compared to PCC, and therefore should only be used if the latter is not available.

In cases where there is no bleeding, management is more conservative and always includes stopping warfarin, with additional therapy dependent on INR:

  i. INR <5: No additional therapy; warfarin may be resumed when INR starts to fall.
  ii. INR 5–9: A small dose of oral vitamin K (1–2.5 mg) can be used, particularly in cases where there is a higher risk of bleeding (e.g. older age, comorbidities), but there is limited evidence to support this.
  iii. INR >9: 2.5–5 mg oral vitamin K should be administered.

In cases of minor bleeding (e.g. low-volume epistaxis) and an elevated INR, warfarin should be held and consideration given to using oral vitamin K, depending on the perceived risk of re-bleeding or progression to major bleeding. It is worth noting that the effect of vitamin K will take 1–2 days, so the INR should be monitored at least daily and further doses given depending on the trend.

Key Points

- Supratherapeutic INR may be due to use of interacting medications, poor compliance with warfarin, dietary variation and acute illness.
- The extent of INR elevation and the presence or absence of bleeding determines the management of a supratherapeutic INR.
- When reversing warfarin effect in patients with major bleeding, prothrombin complex concentrates (Octaplex) should be used in preference to fresh frozen plasma where available.

History

A 54-year-old man receiving immunotherapy for metastatic bladder cancer with known liver and lung metastases presents to the Emergency Department with increasing mid-back pain over the past week. He reports feeling generally weak in his legs, unsteady when he walks, and has been passing urine more frequently than normal.

Examination

Neurologic examination reveals a mildly ataxic gait, with reduced power (3/5 MRC grade) in all muscle groups bilaterally in the lower limbs. There is reduced sensation to light touch ascending from the limbs to just beneath the umbilicus. Knee and ankle reflexes are brisk, and plantar responses are equivocal.

Questions

1. When evaluating a patient with back pain, what are the key features in the history and physical examination that would indicate serious or sinister pathology?
2. What is the likely diagnosis, and what additional clinical information should be elicited?
3. Outline the next steps in managing this patient acutely in the Emergency Department.

DISCUSSION

Acute back pain is not an uncommon reason for presentation to the Emergency Department, and the ability to determine if it requires urgent evaluation and possible admission to the hospital is an important skill. Although the majority of such presentations represent benign pathology, it is important to exclude more serious pathology such as cord or cauda equina compression, infection or abscess. Features in the history warranting greater concern include a prior history of cancer, recent infection or steroid use, fever, pain in the thoracic region, pain that improves with rest and the presence of urinary symptoms. Similarly, 'red flag' examination findings include gait ataxia, generalised weakness, upper motor neurone signs (clonus, hyper-reflexia, extensor plantars), a palpable bladder, saddle anaesthesia and reduced anal tone.

In this case, the history of active cancer together with the neurologic findings point strongly to a diagnosis of malignant spinal cord compression (MSCC). MSCC affects up to 5% of all cancer patients and is the first manifestation of cancer in a fifth of patients. It is more common in cancers that metastasise more frequently to bone, namely prostate, breast, lung and kidney; the majority of bone metastases involve the thoracic (60%) or lumbosacral spine (25%). The presentation of MSCC usually involves increasing pain that is often focal, together with weakness; sensory deficits are seen less frequently, whilst autonomic symptoms (i.e. bladder or bowel dysfunction) occur late in the evolution of MSCC and are a poor prognostic sign.

In this patient, a comprehensive neurologic examination at presentation is paramount, as it will serve as a baseline. It is important to document a sensory level (it appears to be around T11 here so as to guide where one may anticipate abnormalities on imaging). Furthermore, it is important to assess autonomic dysfunction through the history (enquiring about bladder symptoms, urinary retention and incontinence) and examination (looking for saddle anaesthesia and reduced anal sphincter tone).

MSCC is an oncologic emergency, and most institutions have protocols that guide clinicians through the investigations and immediate management when it is suspected. Firstly, radiologic confirmation is required, with the modality of choice being MRI, which carries a sensitivity of 93% and an overall diagnostic accuracy of 95%. A *whole-spine* MRI is required as there may be several levels of compression, some of which may be clinically occult.

Once MSCC is suspected, the patient should receive corticosteroids with gastric protection; typically, IV dexamethasone at a dose between 8 and 16 mg is administered. Further treatment usually involves radiotherapy and/or surgery, with treatment decisions based on prior radiotherapy or surgery, spinal stability, ambulatory status and location of spinal disease. In the rare instances of a highly chemosensitive tumour (e.g. germ cell or lymphoma), upfront chemotherapy may be suitable. Regardless, intensive rehabilitation is required after definitive treatment to maintain and possibly enhance neurologic recovery.

 Key Points

- When evaluating patients with back pain, it is useful to look for 'red flag' symptoms or signs, which indicate serious or sinister pathology.
- Spinal cord compression is an oncologic emergency and usually presents with pain, weakness and sensory deficits.
- Assessment requires careful neurologic examination, including assessment of bladder and bowel function, and imaging by way of whole-spine MRI.

CASE 24: FEELING UNWELL WHILE ON CHEMOTHERAPY

History

A 27-year-old man receiving BEP (bleomycin, etoposide, cisplatin) chemotherapy for testicular cancer presents to the Emergency Department with feeling generally unwell and a self-reported fever. He completed his third and last cycle of chemotherapy 10 days ago and started taking ciprofloxacin 2 days ago as part of his chemotherapy regime.

Examination

Vital signs: temperature of 38.9°C, blood pressure of 90/60, heart rate of 135 and regular, respiratory rate of 28, 95% O_2 saturation on air.

General examination reveals an ill-looking man with cool peripheries. Cardiorespiratory and abdominal examinations are unremarkable, and there is no focal neurology.

 Investigations

- Hb 11.5, WCC 0.4, neutrophils 0.1, PLT 147, Na 132, K 4.2, Ur 7.5, Cr 60.

Questions

1. What are the diagnosis and its underlying pathophysiology?
2. What further assessment and investigations must be performed in the Emergency Department?
3. Outline the key principles in treating this patient.

DISCUSSION

This is a case of neutropaenic sepsis (also known as febrile neutropaenia). Neutropaenic sepsis is defined as a single temperature >38.5°C or two consecutive temperatures >38°C, and an absolute neutrophil count of <0.5 × 10⁹/L or a count <1 × 10⁹/L that is expected to fall. It arises as a result of cytotoxic chemotherapy suppressing the bone marrow, leading to depletion of white blood cells and leaving the individual vulnerable to infection. It is one of the most common complications of cancer therapy, carrying a significant mortality rate of ~5%–10%, and should be regarded as a medical emergency. Any patient receiving chemotherapy and presenting with a fever should be assumed to have neutropaenic sepsis until proven otherwise.

Initial assessment in the Emergency Department should focus on reviewing pertinent aspects of the history, including any prophylactic antibiotic use and prior microbiology results, and examining for potential foci of infection, paying particular attention to any intravascular catheters (e.g. PICC, Hickman) and the mouth (mucositis, which facilitates translocation of bacteria to the bloodstream). It is important to try and avoid breaching skin barriers unless clinically indicated (e.g. performing a digital rectal examination or inserting a urinary catheter) to minimise risk of introducing further infection. Aside from confirming neutropaenia with a full blood count, further investigations required immediately include blood cultures (including culturing each lumen of a central or PICC line if applicable), urine culture and chest radiography as a basic septic screen.

The mainstay of treating neutropaenic sepsis is prompt antibiotic therapy, with international guidelines recommending initiation within 60 minutes of presentation. Choice of antibacterial therapy depends on assessing risk of complications arising from sepsis by utilising instruments such as the Multinational Association for Supportive Care in Cancer (MASCC) index, which scores the severity based on factors such as symptom burden, age, tumour type and presence of hypotension. Lower-risk patients may be treated with oral antibiotics either as an in- or outpatient, whereas higher-risk patients require intravenous therapy as an inpatient. In our patient, the presence of hypotension and cool peripheries point to a high-risk individual requiring inpatient hospitalisation.

Even with appropriate culturing of blood and urine, a specific pathogen may only be identified in up to 20% of cases. Currently, Gram-positive organisms such as *Staphylococci* and *Streptococci* are the most common causes of bacteraemia, having overtaken Gram-negative organisms, particularly *Pseudomonas*, in the past 10–15 years. This is likely as a result of increasing use of long-term indwelling central venous catheters (e.g. Hickman lines or Portacaths) and the inclusion of prophylactic antibiotic therapy within chemotherapy regimes, as is seen in our case.

Antibiotic choice is governed by local guidelines and microbiology resistance patterns, but typically broad-spectrum agents to cover Gram-positive and -negative organisms such as a β-lactam antibiotic (e.g. piperacillin-tazobactam) in combination with an aminoglycoside (e.g. gentamicin) may be used, with addition of other agents in specific circumstances (e.g. vancomycin in case of MRSA positivity). Granulocyte colony-stimulating factors (G-CSF), such as filgrastim, which stimulate production of neutrophils in the bone marrow, are occasionally used as an adjunct particularly in cases where neutropaenia is expected to be prolonged or in individuals at high risk for complications; however, there is little evidence supporting their efficacy, and consensus guidelines recommend against their routine use.

Key Points

- Any cancer patient receiving chemotherapy and presenting a fever should be assumed to have neutropaenic sepsis unless proven otherwise.
- Assessment should focus on identifying a possible infectious source, and performing a prompt septic screen, including taking cultures from peripheral and central veins if appropriate.
- Broad-spectrum antibiotics should be administered within 60 minutes of presentation to a patient with confirmed neutropaenic sepsis and follow locally agreed guidelines.

History

A 70-year-old woman with a 5-day history of worsening cough productive of yellow-green sputum and associated shortness of breath is transferred to the Emergency Department by her General Practitioner. She feels fatigued and has pain when she coughs. She has a history of type 2 diabetes, controlled on metformin, and hypertension, for which she takes amlodipine. She is a non-smoker.

Examination

Vital signs: temperature of 37.8°C, blood pressure of 95/65, heart rate of 90 and regular, respiratory rate of 24, 94% O_2 saturation on air.

General examination reveals a frail-looking woman who is not in acute distress. She is alert and oriented to time, person and place. Cardiac examination is normal, and respiratory examination is notable for crackles at the right base.

Investigations
• Hb 12.4, WCC 14.7 (neutrophils 10.5), PLT 230, Na 138, K 4.5, Ur 9, Cr 75.

Questions

1. What are the differential diagnoses to be considered in this patient? Which diagnosis is most likely?
2. What further investigations should be performed in the Emergency Department, and what treatment would you initiate?
3. Should the patient be admitted to the hospital? Justify your answer.

DISCUSSION

This is a patient presenting with respiratory symptoms (cough with sputum, shortness of breath and chest pain) with localising signs on examination and neutrophilic leucocytosis on laboratory evaluation. The likely diagnoses in this case would include bacterial pneumonia, viral upper or lower respiratory tract infection with or without superadded bacterial infection and pulmonary embolism. Of these, the most likely is a bacterial pneumonia given the presence of purulent sputum and low-grade fever, but there is no clinical prediction tool that can reliably differentiate between viral and bacterial respiratory tract infection, and the diagnosis is largely formed on clinical judgement.

The commonest pathogens that lead to community-acquired pneumonia (CAP) are *Streptococcus pneumoniae*, *Haemophilus influenzae*, *Moraxella catarrhalis* and enteric Gram-negative bacilli; however, a microbiologic diagnosis is only made in about 10% of patients in routine practice. Nevertheless, it would be reasonable to perform limited testing for the pathogen in the ED such as sputum cultures and urine testing for pneumococcal and *Legionella* antigens. A chest radiograph should also be performed as identification of an infiltrate is the gold standard for diagnosing pneumonia; additionally, it may identify evidence of complications, such as cavitation or abscess formation, as well as rule out other lung pathology like a pneumothorax. In terms of treatment, it would be appropriate to fluid-resuscitate this patient given mild hypotension and also to begin empiric antibiotics for CAP. The choice of antibiotics should be based on local guidelines and susceptibilities, but typically includes a beta-lactam to cover *Streptococcus* and a macrolide for atypical coverage.

The decision on whether to hospitalise this patient is tricky, but physicians can use simple scoring systems such as CURB-65 to stratify the severity of CAP. CURB-65 is based upon five easily measurable factors (confusion, urea >7, respiratory rate ≥30, blood pressure <90 systolic or ≤60 diastolic, age ≥65), with a point derived for each factor the patient meets. It has been shown to be predictive of mortality, with a score of 0–1 indicating low severity, with such patients typically managed as an outpatient. A score of 2 or more usually requires admission, with those scoring 3 or more potentially needing intensive care. This patient scores 2 for age and urea, and given that she is mildly hypotensive, has comorbidities and looks frail, she would certainly merit admission to the hospital.

 | **Key Points**

- The common pathogens causing CAP are *S. pneumoniae*, *H. influenzae* and *M. catarrhalis*, but an organism is only found in 10% of cases.
- Always ensure antibiotic coverage for atypical organisms when treating CAP.
- The CURB-65 score can be used to risk-stratify patients and help determine whether they require admission to a hospital.

History

A 52-year-old man is brought to the Emergency Department by an ambulance after suffering from a 'fainting' episode at work. His colleagues noted that he was unsteady on his feet as he stood up from his desk before falling to the ground but did not lose consciousness. He also reports gnawing abdominal pain for the past few hours and vomited dark material on one occasion a few hours earlier. His medical history is notable for chronic back pain, for which he takes 3–4 tablets of ibuprofen daily, and he takes no other prescription medication.

Examination

Vital signs: temperature of 36.5°C, blood pressure of 85/50, heart rate of 125, respiratory rate of 28, 96% O_2 saturation on air.

Physical examination reveals a pale-looking individual who appears in moderate distress. Abdominal examination is notable for epigastric tenderness without rebound or guarding, and digital rectal examination shows black stool.

Investigations
• Hb 8.2, WCC 10.5, PLT 180, lactate 4.5.

Questions

1. What is the likely diagnosis?
2. Outline the first steps in managing this patient in the Emergency Department.
3. How can the patient be risk-stratified, and what is required after his condition is stabilised?

DISCUSSION

This patient presents with a syncopal episode in the setting of likely haematemesis and evidence of melaena on physical examination. These are findings characteristic of an upper gastrointestinal (GI) bleed, with the black stools secondary to breakdown of haemoglobin as blood transits through the GI tract. Important causes of upper GI bleeding include peptic ulcer disease, upper GI malignancy, variceal bleeding in portal hypertension and Mallory–Weiss tears. In this patient, the history of regular use of ibuprofen makes peptic ulcer disease the most likely cause as this, like other non-steroidal anti-inflammatory drugs (NSAIDs), causes gastric mucosal damage by inhibiting production of prostaglandins, which protests the mucosa.

The presence of hypotension and tachycardia indicates moderate–severe blood loss, and the patient should be managed in the resuscitation room. Immediate management should proceed along the 'ABCDE' approach, with consideration of intubation for airway protection in patients with ongoing haematemesis, establishment of at least two sites of large-bore intravenous access and administration of crystalloid fluid boluses. A cross-match should be sent in preparation for possible blood transfusion, and given this patient's hypotension and tachycardia, thereby suggesting active bleeding, at least 1 unit of packed red cells should be transfused with regular monitoring of the haemoglobin. Consideration could even be given to transfusing group O blood given the likely extent of hypovolaemia in this patient. Transfusion is typically performed if the haemoglobin is less than 7 g/dL for most patients, but in cases where active bleeding is suspected, the haemoglobin may be falsely elevated due to haemoconcentration. Proton-pump inhibitors are not recommended pre-endoscopy, but there may be some value in the administration of tranexamic acid, which is currently being evaluated in a large randomised controlled trial (HALTiT).

As the patient is stabilised, urgent consultation with gastroenterology is required in preparation for upper GI endoscopy, particularly in cases of severe bleeding such as this. Risk stratification tools are available to help guide the treating physician on the urgency of endoscopy; the Blatchford score is one such tool and relies on parameters such as the levels of urea and haemoglobin, systolic blood pressure and presence of melaena or syncope. The Rockall score is another such tool, but its use in the emergency setting is hampered by the fact that endoscopic findings are needed in computing the score.

Upper GI endoscopy should be performed once the patient is sufficiently stable, and generally within 24 hours of presentation even in non-severe bleeding. An endoscopy provides both diagnostic and therapeutic benefits, and the findings at endoscopy can also help predict risk of re-bleeding, which is also influenced by other factors such as haemodynamic instability, a haemoglobin of less than 10 g/dL at presentation, large ulcer size and ulcer location. In cases such as this, where several of these factors are present, the patient should ideally be managed in an ICU setting.

 Key Points

- Upper GI bleeding is characterised by haematemesis and melaena, and a history of NSAID use must always be elicited given the associated risk of peptic ulcer disease.
- Supportive management includes fluid resuscitation, blood transfusion (if haemoglobin is <7 g/dL or in cases of active bleeding), intravenous tranexamic acid and preparation for upper GI endoscopy.
- Risk stratification tools such as the Blatchford score can be used to help triage patients and determine the need for an urgent endoscopy.

History

A 35-year-old door-to-door saleswoman is brought in to the Emergency Department by her husband after he thought she had a 'fit' earlier in the day. He reports that she suddenly seemed to lose consciousness, falling to the floor and lying there stiff, before her arms and legs started to jerk. This lasted for about 30 seconds before self-resolving. Afterwards, he realised that she had bitten her tongue and had been incontinent of urine. This episode occurred about 20 minutes ago.

The patient is initially able to open her eyes and speak, but seems sleepy. When obtaining a history, she suddenly loses consciousness and has another similar episode lying stiff and then starts jerking her arms and legs.

Examination

The patient is lying in bed, arms and legs jerking. There is foaming at the mouth.

Questions

1. What is the diagnosis?
2. Describe how you would acutely manage the patient. What would you do if this episode does not self-terminate and has been ongoing for several minutes?
3. Once the patient is stabilised, what investigations should be performed in the ED?

DISCUSSION

This patient's presentation is typical for a generalised tonic–clonic seizure, which is characterised by an abrupt loss of consciousness often accompanied by a loud shriek or shout, followed by a tonic (i.e. muscle contraction, stiffness) and clonic (i.e. muscle relaxation, jerking) phase. During the latter, there may be biting of the tongue or frothy sputum seen coming out of the mouth, as well as loss of bowel or bladder continence. Finally, one of the discriminating features of a seizure is that it is followed by a post-ictal phase with the patient feeling sleepy and only gradually waking up.

Most seizures spontaneously resolve within 1–2 minutes and pharmacotherapy is generally not required. Rather, the aim is to provide supportive care through the seizure (e.g. moving any objects of the patient's way to prevent injury); if the seizure continues beyond 1–2 minutes, a benzodiazepine (4 mg IV lorazepam, 10 mg buccal midazolam or 10–20 mg rectal diazepam) can be administered in an attempt to terminate the episode. Once the seizure has resolved, management should proceed along the 'ABCDE' approach, with airway support and supplementary oxygen administration if needed (e.g. head tilt manoeuvre). Intravenous access should be established, and a point-of-care glucose *must* always be checked as hypoglycaemia is a common cause of seizure.

Status epilepticus is defined as at least 5 minutes of continuous seizures and/or at least two discrete seizure episodes between which consciousness is not fully regained. It is a medical emergency and must always be considered when dealing with a seizing patient. If a patient is suspected of being in status epilepticus, initial assessment and management should focus on securing the airway (with intubation and mechanical ventilation if needed), providing supplemental oxygen to maintain saturation >94% and establishing intravenous access. Emergent investigations should focus on toxic-metabolic causes (i.e. extended electrolytes, glucose, liver function, toxicology, anti-epileptic drug levels), and pharmacologic therapy with benzodiazepines as described above should be initiated with a maximum of two doses. Administration of thiamine and dextrose should be considered, particularly if there is a suspicion for alcohol excess or malnutrition. Concurrently, an infusion of fosphenytoin or phenytoin should be established, with alternatives including sodium valproate or levetiracetam if the patient has intolerance to phenytoin. Metabolic abnormalities should be corrected, but if the patient continues to remain in status epilepticus, expert opinion from Neurology should be obtained and consideration given towards sedation with propofol, midazolam or pentobarbital, and the patient transferred to an intensive care setting.

The ED evaluation of a first seizure should begin with obtaining a thorough history of the episode, both from the patient and any witnesses, paying particular attention to any preceding or triggering events, medication or substance use and family history of seizure disorders. The physical examination should focus on assessing for any localising neurologic signs, and also to evaluate any injuries that the patient may have sustained during the seizure. Key blood tests that need to be checked include those aforementioned, and urine toxicology could be performed to look for substance abuse. An electrocardiogram should be performed, as cardiac syncope may manifest similarly to a seizure, while some form of neuroimaging (CT or MRI) is required in all adults presenting with their first seizure to look for a structural cause. Finally, the decision to pursue specialised testing (lumbar puncture and electroencephalogram [EEG]) is made on a case-by-case basis, with lumbar puncture only done if there is concern for an infectious aetiology and once space-occupying lesions have been excluded, and urgent EEG needed in patients who do not return to their baseline state within 30–60 minutes of the seizure.

Key Points

- Most seizures resolve spontaneously within 1 or 2 minutes, and pharmacotherapy with benzodiazepines is not usually required.
- Status epilepticus is a medical emergency and defined by at least 5 minutes of continuous seizure activity and/or at least two seizure episodes between which consciousness is not fully regained.
- Neuroimaging (with CT or MRI) is mandatory in any adult presenting to the Emergency Department with a first seizure, either on initial presentation or on an urgent outpatient basis.

CASE 28: CHEST PAIN IN A YOUNG WOMAN

History

A 30-year-old woman presents to the Emergency Department with a 2-day history of chest pain. The pain began as a dull and intermittent ache over the left side of her chest and has now progressed to being constant and severe. It is not associated with activity and is not relieved by rest. It is focal in nature and is associated with mild shortness of breath, especially when she tries to take a full breath. She is a non-smoker and there is no family history of cardio-vascular disease.

Examination

Vital signs: temperature of 36.2°C, blood pressure of 120/75, heart rate of 90 and regular, respiratory rate of 16, 96% O_2 saturation on air.

General examination is notable for lack of oedema or distension of the JVP. Cardiac and respiratory examinations are unremarkable, but there is focal tenderness over the medial aspect of the left 4th to 5th ribs. Abdominal examination is normal.

🔍 Investigations

- The electrocardiogram (ECG) is shown below. A chest radiograph shows clear lung fields.

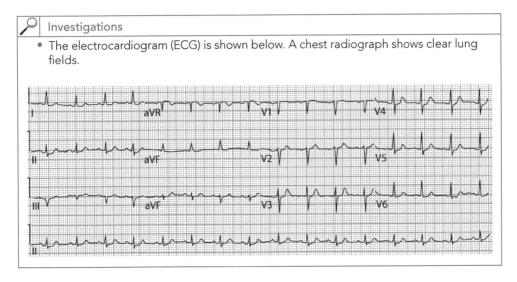

Questions

1. Based on the history and clinical findings, what do you think is the likely diagnosis and why?
2. What investigations would you perform in the ED?
3. Can the patient be discharged from the ED, and should any follow-up be arranged?

DISCUSSION

Chest pain is an extremely common presentation in the ED and can be caused by diseases carrying significant morbidity and mortality, such as myocardial infarction (MI), pulmonary embolism (PE) and aortic dissection. It is therefore crucial that physicians are able to quickly differentiate through the various causes of chest pain and initiate urgent treatment if necessary.

Obtaining a good history forms the basis of evaluating chest pain in the ED. Key features that may help point towards particular diagnoses include

- *Location and radiation* – Central chest pain that radiates to the face, neck or arms is classic for MI, whereas the pain may be more posterior (between shoulder blades) in aortic dissection and unilateral in lung disease.
- *Onset* – Sudden or acute onset pain usually indicates a vascular cause (e.g. PE or aortic dissection), whereas cardiac chest pain is typically more subacute in onset and increases over time.
- *Character* – Cardiac pain is usually described as crushing but may often be a gnawing discomfort, whereas pain associated with aortic dissection and gastrointestinal disorders is usually tearing/ripping and burning, respectively.
- *Exacerbation/alleviation* – Although cardiac pain is typically described as being relieved by administration of a nitrate, this is not a specific indicator as nitrates may also relieve pain from gastrointestinal disorders; however, myocardial ischaemia will manifest as pain brought on by exertion and relieved by rest, which is a good discriminator between cardiac and non-cardiac pain.
- *Associated symptoms* – Shortness of breath, nausea and diaphoresis are frequently noted by patients with MI, while shortness of breath is invariably reported in pulmonary disease; the presence of fever may point towards pneumonia or myocarditis/pericarditis, while syncopal symptoms would be consistent with obstructive cardiac disease (e.g. aortic stenosis) or PE.

Moreover, the history should be placed into the context of the patient's background risk for various diseases (e.g. risk factors such as smoking, diabetes and hypertension would increase likelihood of a cardiac cause; recent long-haul travel or immobility would raise suspicion for PE). Additionally, reviewing the medical record may also be helpful since patients may have recently undergone investigations such as angiography, echocardiography or endoscopy, which may help in focusing the differential diagnosis.

In this case, the patient is young, has no significant cardiac risk factors and has atypical chest pain (non-exertional and not relieved by rest), which makes a cardiac cause very unlikely (it should be noted that the presentation of cardiac disease in women may be more subtle or atypical). The ECG is negative for ischaemia. Pulmonary disease is unlikely as there are no symptoms or signs of PE and no pneumothorax is seen on the chest radiograph; also, there is nothing to suggest an oesophageal cause. Rather, the focal nature of the pain and reproduction of the pain on palpation of the chest wall makes a musculoskeletal cause (e.g. costochondritis) the most likely diagnosis.

The investigations that need to be performed when evaluating chest pain depend largely on the history and clinical suspicion. An ECG is almost always warranted and may suffice in this case; however, it would not be unreasonable to obtain a chest radiograph (to look for any bony abnormalities) and a troponin (a single measurement would rule out MI given the presence of symptoms for 2 days). This patient should be reassured that her pain is unlikely to have a sinister cause, and would be safe to discharge home with advice to take oral analgesics (including NSAIDs) since costochondritis is suspected.

Key Points
• Obtaining a good history is key when evaluating patients with chest pain.
• Always place the history in context of the patient's background and risk factors for various diseases.
• ECG, chest radiograph and blood tests such as troponin and d-dimer should be used to rule out serious causes of chest pain in conjunction with a detailed history.

CASE 29: FAINT IN AN ELDERLY WOMAN

History

An 82-year-old woman is brought to the Emergency Department after fainting in her home. She had been in her kitchen preparing lunch when she suddenly felt light-headed and then passed out. Her husband was with her at the time and reports that she was unconscious for about 10 seconds before regaining it spontaneously. She denies any chest pain before or after the event, and feels well now, albeit a little groggy. She has a history of ischaemic cardiomyopathy, having undergone a triple-vessel CABG more than 10 years ago. Her medications include bisoprolol, amlodipine and lisinopril.

Examination

Vital signs: temperature of 36.5°C, blood pressure of 100/65 (lying) and 95/60 (sitting), heart rate of 45, respiratory rate of 18, 95% O_2 saturation on air.

General examination reveals a well-looking individual who is not in acute distress. Cardiac auscultation is notable for an ejection systolic murmur that radiates to the carotids; the chest is otherwise clear and there is no oedema. Cranial nerve examination is normal.

🔍 **Investigations**

- An electrocardiogram (ECG) is shown below.

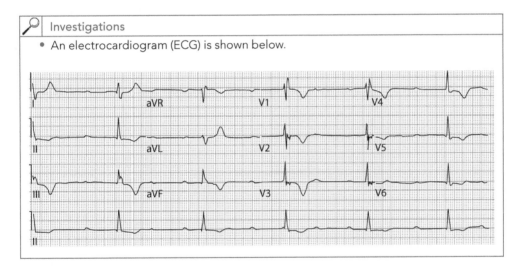

Questions

1. What is the differential diagnosis for syncope?
2. What does the ECG show?
3. Describe how you would manage this patient in the ED. Would your approach change if she had not fainted and the ECG abnormality was picked up incidentally?

DISCUSSION

The history provided in this case fits well with syncope, which refers to transient and self-resolving loss of consciousness that arises as a result of reduced cerebral perfusion. The causes of syncope are often grouped into four categories:

i. *Neurally mediated syncope* – Caused by a reflex response producing bradycardia and/or hypotension (e.g. excessive vagal tone, commonly termed 'vasovagal syncope', which may arise in specific context such as heat, coughing, micturition, etc.)

ii. *Orthostatic syncope* – Defined as a postural decrease in systolic and/or diastolic blood pressures of ≥20 and ≥10 mm Hg, respectively, commonly due to vasodilator medications (e.g. calcium channel blockers) or hypovolaemia

iii. *Cardiac arrhythmia* – This includes both brady- and tachyarrhythmias, notably high-degree atrioventricular (AV) block and ventricular tachycardia

iv. *Structural or obstructive cardiopulmonary disease* – Mediated by reduced cardiac output as a result of blood flow obstruction (e.g. aortic stenosis, pulmonary embolism and acute myocardial infarction)

The differential diagnosis for syncope is seizure, and the two may be distinguished by the absence of a quick or spontaneous recovery with a seizure, where a post-ictal state (sleepiness, confusion, lethargy) is present.

In this patient, the ECG shows evidence of complete heart block, with p waves and QRS complexes occurring independently of each other. The result is a junctional escape rhythm, which leads to bradycardia and syncope. Potential causes of complete heart block in this patient include chronic ischaemic damage to the conducting system and medication-related AV block from bisoprolol and/or amlodipine.

Management of this patient should proceed along the Advanced Life Support (ALS) bradycardia algorithm. She should be placed on a cardiac monitor in the resuscitation room and blood should be drawn to check for electrolytes (including potassium, calcium and magnesium), as severe metabolic disturbance can lead to bradycardia. Seeing as she presented with syncope and remains bradycardic, 500 µg atropine should be given, and can be repeated every few minutes to a total dose of 3 mg. Her rate and rhythm should be assessed frequently, with consideration given to transthoracic pacing or an isoprenaline infusion if she does not respond. Cardiology input should be sought, as she will likely require a transvenous pacemaker given the risk of asystole associated with high-grade AV block. In the event that she did not present symptomatically with syncope (or other 'high-risk' features such as shock, myocardial ischaemia or hypotension), management would remain the same due to presence of complete heart block. Observation would only be appropriate if she did *not* present with high-risk features *and* her rhythm was *not* one associated with a high risk for asystole (i.e. ventricular pause >3 seconds, Mobitz type II AV block, complete heart block or recent episode of asystole). In such cases, it would be worth addressing reversible causes of bradycardia (e.g. toxicity from beta-blockers), but input should still be sought from cardiology either in the ED or at outpatient follow-up.

Key Points

- Syncope is a transient loss of consciousness arising as a result of reduced perfusion to the brain.
- Atropine should be used in symptomatic bradycardia as well as bradycardia associated with high-risk rhythms such as Mobitz type II block.
- Always involve cardiology in patients with symptomatic bradycardia as a pacemaker may be urgently required.

CASE 30: AN ABNORMAL ECG

History

A 56-year-old man is found lying alone on a park bench next to several bottles of whisky and brought into the Emergency Department due to concerns about his safety. He is not able to provide much history but reports that he has been experiencing worsening abdominal pain and bloating for the past few days. His medical history is notable for alcoholism with associated cirrhosis and cardiomyopathy, but he presents infrequently for medical appointments and is non-compliant with medications. He drinks heavily and has done so for several years.

Examination

Vital signs: temperature of 37.6°C, blood pressure of 100/60, heart rate of 125 and irregular, respiratory rate of 18, 93% O$_2$ saturations on air.

General examination reveals an unkempt individual with evidence of asterixis and stigmata of chronic liver disease. Heart sounds are present with no murmurs, but the rhythm is irregular. Abdominal examination reveals a distended abdomen, and shifting dullness and a fluid thrill are noted. Abbreviated Mental Test Score is 6/10.

🔍 Investigations

- An electrocardiogram (ECG) is performed (see below). A previous ECG from 2 years ago showed normal sinus rhythm.

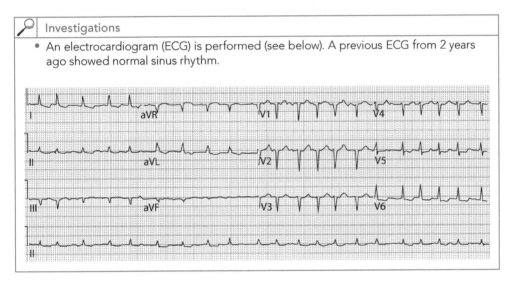

Questions

1. What does the ECG show? What do you suspect precipitated this and why?
2. What investigations should be performed in the ED?
3. How would you manage this patient acutely, and what would you consider when making decisions on treatment?

DISCUSSION

The ECG shows an irregularly irregular rhythm with no evidence of P waves, as well as tachycardia, consistent with atrial fibrillation (AF) with rapid ventricular rate, colloquially known as 'fast AF'. AF is the commonest cardiac arrhythmia and is frequently encountered in the ED as well as in inpatient wards. It arises as a result of ectopic atrial activity from sites other than the sinoatrial node, with not all beats being captured by the ventricles, thereby leading to an irregular rate and lack of P waves on the ECG. It is associated with several conditions, including structural and valvular heart disease, ischaemic heart disease, cardiomyopathy, obstructive lung disease, metabolic disorders (e.g. hyperthyroidism), electrolyte abnormalities (e.g. hypokalaemia, hypomagnesaemia) and acute illness (e.g. sepsis, postoperative state). This patient has a history of alcoholism and findings consistent with alcoholic cirrhosis and therefore likely has some degree of alcoholic cardiomyopathy, thereby predisposing him to development of AF. An additional trigger may be his acute illness, with the evidence of a low-grade fever and abdominal pain in a patient with ascites pointing towards possible spontaneous bacterial peritonitis (SBP).

The initial evaluation of this patient should include checking a full blood count, electrolytes including magnesium, clotting screen, thyroid function and a chest radiograph. If there were suspicion for cardiac ischaemia or heart failure, it would be reasonable to check cardiac enzymes and a BNP. A transthoracic echo should also be arranged but is not required emergently. In this patient, an ascitic tap should also be performed to look for SBP.

The acute management of the patient should proceed along the 'ABCDE' approach, with delivery of supplemental oxygen (given saturation of <94% on air). The patient appears to be relatively haemodynamically stable despite the tachycardia, and therefore heart rate control would be warranted, with the aim to control rates to 110 or less. This can be achieved through use of calcium channel blockers or beta-blockers (e.g. IV diltiazem infusion or IV metoprolol boluses, followed by oral medication); digoxin may also be used, particularly in patients with evidence or history of heart failure.

The other treatment approach in patients with AF is restoration of sinus rhythm via electrical or chemical cardioversion. Electrical (DC) cardioversion should be performed emergently in patients with AF who are unstable (e.g. hypotension, evidence of heart failure or organ hypoperfusion), but the downside is that cardioversion may lead to systemic embolisation of a left atrial thrombus, assuming that the patient has had AF for a sustained period of time. If it can be confidently assumed that the patient has been in AF for less than 48 hours (i.e. via documentation of rhythm through ECGs or symptoms), cardioversion is appropriate, but it should otherwise be deferred until a transoesophageal echocardiogram is performed to confirm the absence of atrial thrombus or until the patient has been anti coagulated for a period of at least 3 weeks. In this case, it is quite likely that the patient has had AF for a reasonable period of time given the likelihood of alcoholic cardiomyopathy, and since there is no evidence that AF is new onset, cardioversion should be deferred in favour of rate control unless he became unstable.

The final consideration in patients with AF is anticoagulation, as they are at risk for systemic embolisation and stroke (due to stasis of blood in the left atrium). This can be assessed through use of the CHADSVASC and HASBLED scores, which predict risk of thrombosis without anticoagulation and bleeding, respectively.

Key Points

- An irregularly irregular rhythm with an absence of P waves on the ECG is consistent with atrial fibrillation (AF).
- AF with rapid ventricular rates is generally managed with control of heart rates through use of beta-blockers or calcium-channel blockers.
- Unstable patients with AF may require electrical cardioversion to restore sinus rhythm.

History

A 40-year-old man presents to the Emergency Department with a history of episodic high fever and feeling generally unwell. He returned 1 week ago from a 10-day holiday to rural Assam, India, where he was visiting his family. He received his required travel vaccinations before the trip but did not take any antimalarial prophylaxis. Other family members who travelled with him have not reported similar symptoms. He has a history of asthma, which is controlled with inhalers, and is a non-smoker.

Examination

Vital signs: temperature of 38.2°C, blood pressure of 105/70, heart rate of 90 and regular, respiratory rate of 20, 95% O_2 saturation on air.

He is not in acute distress, and his extremities are warm and well-perfused. There is no rash or evidence of meningism. Cardiac, respiratory and abdominal examinations are unremarkable.

Questions

1. What additional history should be obtained from the patient in the Emergency Department?
2. What is the differential diagnosis? Which diagnoses are more likely, given the travel history?
3. What initial investigations are you going to perform?

DISCUSSION

Up to 1 in 10 travellers seek medical advice for various symptoms after returning home from a trip. Fever is a very common symptom in returning travellers and has a broad differential diagnosis, ranging from life-threatening to self-limiting illness. Therefore, such patients need a systematic evaluation that aims to elucidate not only whether an infectious disease is the cause but also whether that disease is transmissible, as this has important public health implications.

Key aspects of the history that should be gathered in this case include

- Geographic details about the countries and specific locations visited on the trip, dates of the trip, whether the patient was predominantly in a rural or urban area, and where they stayed (e.g. hotel or local accommodation)
- Activities and potential exposures during travel, such as sexual contacts, needle and blood exposure, insect or mosquito bites, contact with animals or animal products (e.g. rodents, bats) and type of food and beverages consumed (e.g. tap water, unpasteurised milk)
- Host factors that may predispose to infections, including immunocompromised state (e.g. HIV, splenectomy), vaccine history, use of antimicrobial prophylaxis (e.g. malaria), past medical/infectious history and illness in fellow travellers

The differential diagnosis of fever in this returning traveller is broad, with the commonest diagnoses including malaria, viral fevers (dengue, chikungunya), viral mononucleosis (EBV, CMV), typhoid and viral hepatitis. Other differentials include non-specific viral infections, influenza, bacterial skin or soft tissue infections (*Staphylococcus* or *Streptococcus*), urinary tract infection, bacterial pneumonia and tuberculosis. The possibility of acute HIV infection should also be considered, particularly if there are risk factors such as new sexual contact or blood exposure.

Of these conditions, the most likely diagnosis in this patient would be malaria, given that it is endemic in parts of India, commonly presents with fever alone as a symptom in contrast to other conditions where there may be other localising symptoms or signs, and no anti-malarial prophylaxis was taken prior to or during the trip.

The initial evaluation of this patient in the Emergency Department should include obtaining basic blood tests (full blood count, electrolytes, liver function, clotting screen), blood cultures, urinalysis and a chest radiograph. Blood films for malaria are crucial and should include both thick and thin films to screen for parasites, and quantify parasitaemia and to identify the malarial species, respectively. These should be repeated if initially negative. There are also rapid diagnostic tests, which test for malarial antigens, and these can also be used if locally available. Additional testing should be performed based on clinical suspicion (e.g. serology for dengue or chikungunya, hepatitis serologies, or stool cultures for diarrhoeal disease), but would not be necessarily indicated in this patient unless baseline blood testing revealed other abnormalities such as deranged liver function. It is also important to alert the local public health authorities should malaria testing be positive, as it is a notifiable disease.

Key Points

- Taking a thorough travel and exposure history is crucial when evaluating unwell returning travellers in the Emergency Department.
- The differential diagnosis of fever in a returning traveller includes malaria, viral fevers, acute HIV infection, typhoid and viral hepatitis.
- Always perform thick and thin blood films to test for malaria in travellers who have been to malaria-endemic regions.

History

A 23-year-old man has returned from Vietnam 2 days ago and presents to the Emergency Department. He complains of high fevers, mild headache and copious loose stools with traces of blood. He travelled through both urban and rural areas on a cycling holiday and was keen to sample the local food and enjoy the nightlife. As this trip was last-minute, he did not have time for any vaccinations or any anti-malarials.

Examination

The patient appears to be comfortable at rest but looks dehydrated clinically. There is a rash over the top half of his torso and abdomen. The abdomen is soft with generalised vague tenderness. Digital rectal examination reveals an empty rectum with a trace of blood. Cardiovascular, respiratory and nervous system examinations are normal apart from a resting bradycardia.

Vitals signs reveal: temperature of 39.2°C, blood pressure of 120/70, heart rate of 58 and regular, respiratory rate of 20, 97% O_2 saturation on air.

 Investigations
- Venous blood gas: pH 7.21, Na 130, K 2.8, Cl 90, HCO_3 20, BE -4.8, lactate 3.0

Questions
1. What is the likely diagnosis?
2. How are you going to investigate this patient?
3. What are potential complications?

DISCUSSION

This patient has signs and symptoms of dysentery following a trip abroad. Dysentry is defined as diarrhoea with blood. The initial assessment for travellers should start with a detailed history. This should encompass travel plans, vaccinations and prophylactic medications. Care should be taken to plot the entire journey including any stopovers in other countries. The history should be full and detailed and include the onset of any prodromal symptoms and the time of onset of the current illness. Patients should be asked about their activities whilst on holiday including adventurous trips to rural areas and about their food habits and hygiene. You should also ask if any travelling companions are unwell and if the patient sought any treatment on holiday including self-prescribed or over-the-counter medications. It is possible to buy antibiotics and other medications in developing countries without prescription. You should also take a sexual history.

Investigation of the returned traveller requires a systematic approach as tests will need to be tailored to the clinical presentation and suspected diagnosis. It would be prudent to perform basic blood tests including a full blood count, renal function, liver function, amylase, C-reactive protein and malarial screen as a starting point in the ED. A chest radiograph should also be considered to rule out an atypical pneumonia and HIV and hepatitis screening offered particularly if the patient is high-risk (the systemic illness may be due to HIV seroconversion). Care should be taken to rule out 'non-tropical' causes such as appendicitis or meningitis by clinical examination and history.

The most likely diagnosis for this patient is typhoid fever. There is the presence of systemic fever, bloody diarrhoea and a rash referred to as 'rose' spots. The key in this case is the relative bradycardia in the presence of hypovolaemia and fever. Although the patient is physically fit as suggested by the cycling holiday, this is typical of typhoid fever. Typhoid fever is caused by either *Salmonella typhi or Salmonella paratyphi* and is endemic throughout Southeast Asia, India, Africa and South America. Clinical symptoms start between 7 and 21 days from infection. It is typically acquired by the faeco-oral route and associated with poor hand hygiene or contaminated food from local or 'street' sources. It often has an insidious onset compared to other causes of gastroenteritis, and symptoms may occur over a few days to weeks. Initial diagnosis may be clinical as in this case, and it is often picked up in stool samples in returned travellers sent either via their GP or via the Emergency Department.

This patient will need inpatient treatment as he is dehydrated and the venous blood gas suggests an early acute kidney injury and hypokalaemia. He will need intravenous rehydration and then treatment with either ciprofloxacin, ceftriaxone or azithromycin for between 7 and 14 days. Anti-microbial advice should be sought as fluoroquinolone-resistant strains exist.

Other possible causes of dysentery include *E. coli*, *Shigella*, *Campylobacter* and *Yersinia*. They all present with similar illnesses, and the only reliable way to differentiate them is on stool culture. Giardia or amoebic dysentery is less likely as this is associated with less systemic upset and more explosive diarrhoea and borborygmi. There is also the possibility of parasitic worm infection, and stool samples should be sent for ova, cyst and parasite screening. Eosinophilia on full blood count testing may also support a diagnosis of parasitic worm infection.

Typhoid fever is associated with complications such as intestinal perforation, myocarditis and meningitis. Surgical consultations should be obtained if complications are suspected.

This patient will need repeat stool testing after treatment as there can be chronic carriage in the gallbladder. Eradication is achieved with a prolonged (28 days) course of antibiotics. It is also a 'notifiable' disease, and patients should be encouraged not to return to work whilst they are unwell especially if they work with food or in a public organisation such as a school. Unwell travelling companions should undergo assessment and treatment as necessary.

The best form of protection for travellers is vaccination prior to travel. As this trip was planned at short notice, the patient was not vaccinated and so was at higher risk whilst on holiday. An oral live vaccine and an injectable polysaccharide coat vaccine are commonly used, with the injectable form favoured in the United Kingdom (Typhim or Typherix Vi).

 Key Points

- A comprehensive travel history is important when assessing fever in the returned traveller.
- Investigations should be tailored to the clinical presentation and likely diagnoses.
- Typhoid fever may need prolong antibiotics for complete eradication.
- Salmonella infections are a public health risk, and the patient should be encouraged not to return to work until completion of treatment.

MENTAL HEALTH AND OVERDOSE

CASE 33: UNCONSCIOUS JOHN DOE

History

A 46-year-old man is brought in to the Emergency Department by police officers, having been found in the street. Police officers report he was lying still and appeared inactive next to several cans of beer and vomitus. The patient is not carrying any identity and unable to give you any further history.

Examination

Vital signs: temperature of 36.2°C, blood pressure of 145/86, heart rate of 99 and regular, respiratory rate of 10, 94% O_2 saturations on air.

You note an unkempt gentleman, with a strong smell of urine and alcohol, snoring loudly on the hospital bed. There is bilateral air entry, with crackles at both bases. Heart sounds are normal. He appears drowsy but rousable (GCS E3, V2, M5). Glucose is 4.2 mmol/L.

Questions

1. What is your differential diagnosis?
2. What is your initial management?
3. How will you clinically assess the severity of this patient's condition?
4. How would you further manage this patient?

DISCUSSION

Alcohol is the most commonly overused toxin presenting to the Emergency Department. In the United Kingdom, the National Institute on Alcohol Abuse and Alcoholism reports rising trends in the use of alcohol in people aged 18 years or older, with an estimated 25% reporting they engage in binge drinking and 7% reporting heavy drinking in the past month.

There are several alcohols that are available to the public over the counter: ethanol, methanol, ethylene glycol (found in coolants and antifreeze) and isopropyl alcohol (found in solvents and hand sanitisers). The most common alcohol, ethanol, is primarily metabolised by the liver via the alcohol dehydrogenase pathway to form acetaldehyde, which is then further metabolised by acetaldehyde dehydrogenase to form acetate. The redox reaction requires NAD^+ as a cofactor, resulting in the rise of the $NADH/NAD^+$ ratio in the cytosol. This results in alcohol-related complications e.g. hypoglycaemia, hyperlactaemia, inhibition of Krebs cycle and steatosis.

Acute ethanol intoxication presents initially with disinhibition, followed by euphoria. Imbibing large amounts of ethanol can result in acute gastritis, which is characterised by epigastric pain, and vomiting. However, further ingestion can result in in-coordination, ataxia, stupor and coma. The latter can result in accidental injury, in particular head injury and respiratory depression resulting in aspiration or respiratory arrest.

Differentials that may mimic acute alcohol intoxication include

- Hypoglycaemia
- Electrolyte disturbance
- Vitamin depletion (B12/folate)
- Head trauma
- Sepsis
- Other toxins or drug overdose
- Other causes for CNS depression

An airway assessment, neurological examination and survey for accidental injury are required. In particular, to exclude other causes for reduced levels of consciousness. Signs of chronic liver disease or infection should also be noted and managed.

Furthermore, a detailed alcohol history is vital to assess risk of two serious, yet preventable, complications of alcohol cessation – delirium tremens and acute Wernicke's encephalopathy. Tools such a CIWA-Ar are useful in the assessment and management of acute alcohol withdrawal. Screening tools (e.g. Short Alcohol Dependence Data Questionnaire, Alcohol Use Disorder Identification Test, Fast Alcohol Screening Test) are useful in assessing patients at risk of alcohol dependency and should be performed on all patients.

Patients should undergo blood tests to rule out acute or chronic disturbances including a full blood count, electrolytes (including phosphate, calcium and magnesium), vitamin B12, folate, liver enzymes and amylase. Glucose should be checked and hypoglycaemia should be corrected. Thiamine should also be supplemented in those who have alcohol dependence. Patient that are considered to be alcohol dependent may develop delirium tremens and thus require monitoring (see Table 33.1).

If the patient recovers from the acute episode, appearing alert, with stable vital signs, it may be an opportunity to take a further medical and psychiatric history. Consider discharge with

Table 33.1 **Signs and management for delirium tremens**

Signs	Management
Coarse tremor, agitation, cognitive impairment, psychosis	Vitamin supplements
	• Vitamin B
Sweating, tachycardia	• Thiamine
Tonic–clonic seizure	• Vitamin C
Fever might also be present	Correct hypoglycaemia
	Correct hypophosphataemia
	Long-acting benzodiazepine; in severe cases, can consider IM haloperidol

follow-up with the psychiatric or medical team if appropriate. Refer the patient to the alcohol rehabilitation program.

If the patient is at high risk of alcohol withdrawal, stupor or coma, they should be admitted. Regular vitamin supplements and long-acting benzodiazepine should be given to minimise risk of acute Wernicke's encephalopathy or delirium tremens.

 Key Points

- Concurrent physical injuries can occur with acute alcohol intoxication, and a full examination should be performed if a patient is not able to offer a full medical history.
- Most patients only require supportive treatment.
- Once recovered, the patient should receive psychiatric assessment if there is suspicion of intentional overdose.
- Consider admitting the patient to a hospital if he or she develops worrying symptoms and signs of acute alcohol withdrawal.

History

A 19-year-old male is brought in to the Emergency Department in a critical condition after his family found him to be confused. The patient's father reports that he found empty packets of medications in his son's room including an antidepressant. The patient has no known allergies or significant past medical history. His parents mentioned that he has recently been keeping to himself, not attending university classes or socialising with friends. He was known to be very bright, but also had failed his recent mid-year exams.

Examination

Vital signs: temperature of 38.2°C, blood pressure of 146/90, heart rate of 110 and regular, respiratory rate of 10, 92% O_2 saturation on air.

The patient is grunting on the hospital trolley, disorientated in space and time and not responding to commands. His pupils are dilated and his mouth is very dry. Bowel sounds are quiet, with dullness to percussion in the suprapubic area.

 Investigations

- The electrocardiogram shows a sinus rhythm with widened QRS complexes and a QTc of 540 ms.

Questions

1. What important factors in the history should be elicited?
2. What drug overdose syndrome is presented in this case?
3. What are the next steps in the management of this patient?

DISCUSSION

The history and examination findings in this patient are suggestive of a tricyclic antidepressant overdose (Table 34.1). Over 50% of suicidal overdoses involve more than one medication and are often taken with alcohol. History and examination are often limited on arrival, and so initial management of suspected overdoses can be approached with the following five steps:

Step 1: Support. All patients presenting acutely should be assessed and managed using the 'ABCDE' approach – in this case, fluids, cooling and short-acting benzodiazepines to control agitation. History, if possible, should evaluate possible toxins implicated (time of ingestion and quantity) and if there are any known patient medical history or allergies. Most drugs result in acid–base imbalance, and therefore primary investigations should include urea and electrolytes, lactate and blood gas (acid–base deficit should be calculated).

Step 2: Decontaminate. The next step will involve reducing absorption of suspected exposure; this can be achieved through skin decontamination or oral administration of activated charcoal.

Activated charcoal is a carbon-rich substance that is usually processed to increase the surface area. The aim of oral ingestion is to bind to the toxin, thereby reducing ingestion. It is usually indicated in the first hour of ingestion, however, and can be given if the suspected drug has low lipid solublility, has slow release or has a slow transit time. However, activated charcoal is relatively ineffective for heavy metals, pesticides, alcohols, cyanide or strong acids/alkalis, which do not bind to its surface. It can cause vomiting and is thus not suitable for patients that are unable to protect their airway or if strong chemicals were ingested, as they may cause oesophageal perforation or severe chemical pneumonitis. Activated charcoal can be combined with laxative such as Klean-Prep, which contains a strong osmotic agent (macrogol) with a balanced electrolyte solution to increase gastrointestinal transit, thereby further limiting absorption of the toxin. Large fluid loss can result of the cleansing resulting in renal dysfunction.

Alternatively, gastric lavage can be performed to empty the contents of the stomach. This is not often performed due to high risk of aspiration and not favoured by patients, and is thus reserved if time of ingestion is <1 hour, and fatal doses of toxins are suspected.

Step 3: Eliminate. The aim of elimination is to remove the toxin safely from circulations, and can be achieved in certain circumstances using the following methods: urinary alkalinisation, haemodialysis or haemoperfusion.

Urinary alkanisation enhances excretion of weak acid and is useful if moderate salicylate poisoning is suspected. Emergency haemodialysis may be indicated based on following criteria (Table 34.2). Patients not responding to medical management, yet not meeting strict criteria, should be discussed with HDU/ITU or the renal team (as per local pathways). Haemoperfusion is an alternate therapy that utilises an extracorporeal circuit (often contains components of charcoal, or alternate resin) to absorb toxins. However, similarly to oral activated charcoal, haemoperfusion may provide limited benefit in alcohol, pesticides, heavy metals, cyanide, strong acids or alkali poisoning.

Table 34.1 Clinical syndromes that have been recognised due to elevated level of toxins

Toxin	RR	HR and BP	Temp	Pupil	Bowel sound	Diaphoresis	Other
Anticholinergic, e.g. antidepressants, antihistamines	–	Increased	Increased	Mydriasis	Reduced	Reduced	Urinary retention, confusion
Cholinergic, e.g. organophosphates, carbamate	–	–	–	Miosis	Increased	Increased	Increased bronchial secretion, lacrimation
Sympathomimetic, e.g. cocaine, amphetamine	Increased	Increased	Increased	Mydriasis	Increased	Increased	Intracerebral bleeds, seizures
Opiate (morphine)	Reduced	Reduced	Reduced	Miosis	Reduced	Reduced	Coma
Sedative-hypnotic, e.g. anticonvulsants, benzodiazepine	Reduced	Reduced	Reduced	–	Reduced	Reduced	Ataxia, diplopia, nystagmus, apnea

Note: BP = blood pressure; HR = heart rate; RR = respiratory rate; Temp = temperature.

Table 34.2 Criteria for consideration of haemodialysis

- Fluid retention leading to pulmonary oedema, not responding to diuretics
- Hyperkalaemia (>6.5 mmol/L) and not responding to medical management
- Severe acid–base disturbance (pH <7.0)
- Ureaemia (urea >30 mmol/L, creatinine >500 μmol/L) or clinical signs such as pericarditis, neuropathy or enecephalopathy
- Toxin amenable to dialysis (salicylates, ethylene glycol, methanol, lithium, phenobarbital)

Table 34.3 Antidote to common poisons/toxins

Poison	Reversal agent
Paracetamol	Acetylcysteine, methionine
Opiates	Naloxone
Benzodiazepine	Flumazenil
β-blockers	Glucagon
Tricyclic antidepressent	Sodium bicarbonate
Calcium channel blockers	Calcum gluconate or calcium chloride
Carbon monoxide	Oxygen (hyperbaric)
Digoxin	Digoxin specific antibodies
Ethylene glycol, methanol	Ethanol, fomepizole
Organophosphates	Atropine, pralidoxime
Cyanide	Dicobalt edetate, hydroxocobalamin, sodium nitrate

Step 4: Reverse. Once we have considered reducing absorption, and eliminating toxin from circulation, we can now consider reversing the effects of the toxin. Table 34.3 gives an example of common poison and antidotes; however, the list is not exhaustive. Most Emergency Departments in the United Kingdom register to a toxicology service (e.g. TOXBASE), and it is advisable to follow up-to-date advice on managing acute poisoning.

Step 5: Refer. Finally, all patients with acute poisoning, once stable, should undergo psychiatric assessment, especially if deliberate self-harm is suspected.

Consider admission to a general medical or Emergency Department observation unit if the patient is asymptomatic, but the known drug has a potentially life-threatening delayed reaction (e.g. aspirin, paracetamol, lithium, tricyclic antidepressants or if the drug taken is slow or has modified release formulation). The patient should be observed if he or she develops concerning symptoms such as respiratory depression, palpitation or dizziness. Mild gastrointestinal upset is expected in most cases.

The National Poisons Information Service (NPIS) provides assistance, and it is advisable to contact them if considering discharge of a high-risk individual (social concerns, elderly or young, lives alone).

Alternatively, unstable patients should be referred to intensive care if they

- Are haemodynamically unstable
- Have an altered mental state or inability to protect airway
- Have seizures following drug ingestion

Key Points

- Most toxins can be managed safely with first principles of the Emergency Department – Support, Decontaminate, Eliminate, Reverse and Refer.
- Consider ITU admission or renal replacement therapy in patients with extreme acid–base imbalance or those requiring respiratory support.
- Patients should receive psychiatric assessment once stable.

History

A 21-year-old girl is brought to the Emergency Department by her friend, having been found to have taken a paracetamol overdose. Her friend reports she took 48 tablets of paracetamol (500 mg) 2 days ago, with a bottle of vodka. Subsequently, she has vomited several times and was complaining of severe abdominal tenderness. She is now drowsy and unable to give you a further history.

Examination

Vital signs: temperature of 35.6°C, blood pressure of 114/62, heart rate of 100 and regular, respiratory rate of 30, 100% O_2 saturations on air.

Physical examination reveals a drowsy slim female who appears to maintain her own airway. Capillary refill time is >3 seconds, and she is clammy to touch. Blood glucose is 2.1 mmol/L. Pupils are equal and reactive to light. She groans when palpating her upper right quadrant of her abdomen; there is no bruising.

 Investigations

- An arterial blood gas (on room air) shows pH 7.13, pO_2 10.2, pCO_2 3.0, HCO_3 10.

Questions

1. What is the pathophysiology of paracetamol toxicity?
2. How would you initially manage the patient?
3. When would you consider referral to a specialist liver unit?

DISCUSSION

In the setting of drug overdose, paracetamol is the common medication of choice. Most patients presenting acutely are asymptomatic or complain of mild abdominal symptoms such as nausea and vomiting. Without correction, this may progress to severe vomiting and hepatic tenderness. Late signs of liver failure may become more apparent several days after the insult. This includes hepatic encephalopathy, jaundice, hypoglycemia, renal failure, metabolic acidosis and coagulopathy.

In the acute setting, it is important to ascertain amount ingested and its timing. In usual doses, active paracetamol is conjugated in the liver to its inactive form; a small percentage is metabolised by cytochrome P450 to produce the toxic metabolite N-acetyl–p–benzoquinone (NAPQI), which is inactivated by undergoing further conjugation with glutathione. As the paracetamol levels rise, a greater percentage of paracetamol is metabolised by the cytochrome P450 pathway, resulting in higher levels of NAPQI. Hepatic necrosis occurs once the reserves of glutathione are diminished and no mechanism is then available to dispose NAPQI. This usually occurs at levels >150 mg/kg. Risk factors for hepatic toxicity include a history of chronic alcohol misuse, malnutrition, cystic fibrosis and HIV. The latter has reduced glutathione reserves and is at greater risk of NAPQI production, and thus hepatic toxicity.

Initial blood investigations should include liver function tests, INR (clotting screen), renal function tests (including creatinine and electrolytes) and a venous blood gas analysis to check bicarbonate and metabolic acidosis. Blood paracetamol levels should be checked 4 hours after ingestion, ideally before the administration of N-acetylcysteine (NAC). Liver function tests and INR, which may remain normal in the acute setting, may subsequently deteriorate over the next few days. These are also important prognostic markers of severity and function of liver injury.

Patients who have taken a single acute overdose of paracetamol over less than 1 hour should be given NAC (Parvolex) if their plasma paracetamol concentration is above the normogram (see Figure 35.1). All patients who have taken doses of paracetamol staggered over more than

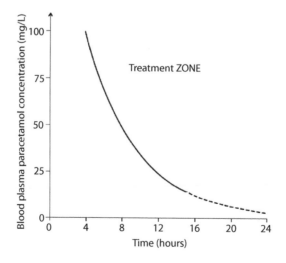

Figure 35.1 Paracetamol treatment normogram. Patient blood concentration should be checked after at least 4 hours of ingestion. Treatment should be started if the concentration of paracetamol is above the treatment line.

1 hour should be treated with NAC as per the Commission on Human Medicine (CHM) advice. Other patients who require consideration for the immediate administration of NAC are those who have ingested >150 mg/kg/24 hours; if there is uncertainty about the timing or amount of ingestion; jaundice; or liver tenderness.

Patients should be monitored for side effects of NAC, which include erythema, urticaria, bronchospasm, angioedema and hypotension. An alternative to NAC is methionine, which can be given orally if intravenous access is not possible.

Patients meeting the following criteria should be referred to an acute liver unit for consideration of a liver transplant:

1. pH <7.3
2. Prothrombin time >100 seconds
3. Creatinine >300 μmol/L
4. Lactate >3.5 mmol/L on admission or >3.0 mmol/L despite fluid resuscitation
5. Grade 3 or higher hepatic encephalopathy

Stable patients should be referred to an acute psychiatric service for further assessment of self-harm/suicidal ideation.

 Key Points

- Paracetamol poisoning is the most common overdose presentation, and it is important to evaluate the amount taken and method (single or staggered overdose).
- N-acetylcysteine treatment should be monitored due to risk of bronchospasm, angioedema and hypotension.
- All patients should receive a psychiatric assessment once stable.
- Severe metabolic acidosis (pH <7.3), deranged clotting, acute kidney injury and acute cognitive impairment are negative prognostic markers and may warrant referral to a specialist liver unit.

CASE 36: ATTEMPTED SUICIDE

History

A 54-year-old man is brought to the Emergency Department by ambulance. He had attempted to slit the left side of his throat with a knife. The patient stated he 'had enough' and 'there is absolute no way out'. He recently lost a large sum of money to a fraudster. He is a full-time carer for his mother, who has advanced dementia.

He explained that it was a spur of the moment suicide attempt. He knew that he had not cut deep enough. He had sent text messages to a close friend prior to attempting suicide.

He studied psychology at university and says he worked in an administration job until about 10 years ago. He has no children or other family. He has no history of mental or physical health problems, or any forensic history. He does not smoke or drink alcohol, and denies illicit drug use.

He states his father suffered from depression and committed suicide by hanging himself several years ago.

Examination

Examination reveals a disheveled-looking man, who avoids eye contact. He has a superficial 5 cm laceration on the left side of his neck. He is alert, oriented and responsive.

Questions

1. How would you perform a suicide risk assessment?
2. What investigations would you perform?
3. Would you admit this patient to the hospital, and if so, why?

DISCUSSION

Self-harm and attempted suicide are distressing for all involved. Over the past decade, there has been a substantial increase in the incidence of self-harm and suicide, especially amongst men aged 11–16 years. Intentional self-harm results in around 150,000 attendances to the ED. These patients are 100 times more likely to commit suicide within the next year compared to the general population.

Self-harm and suicide are often used interchangeably, but are in fact two separate entities. Suicide is a self-inflicted intentional act to cause death, whereas self-harm is a complex behaviour to inflict harm but not associated with the thought of dying – a method to relieve mental stress by inflicting physical pain.

Firstly, a patient's mental capacity, willingness to participate in consultation and any pre-existing mental health history should be assessed, as this will govern further management. Patients should be deemed to have capacity, unless there is strong evidence of cognitive impairment – such as a primary underlying diagnosis of dementia, or induced by toxins or in emergency life-threatening scenario. All patients should be managed with the same dignity and respect as non-self-harming patients. Their physical injury should be managed regardless of their willingness to participate in psychological assessment. As the event can be distressing, the patient should be kept in a safe environment.

In the history, try to obtain as much detail about the patient (birth, education, employment and social relations) – in particular, focusing on the potential risk factors (Table 36.1) and red flags (Table 36.2). Take a timeline of events and the circumstances around the event, and evaluate how much planning went into the act, if the patient was intending to be found or not. Also, enquire about the length of time they contemplated over the act, previous acts of self-harm and if they escalated the severity of the acts. Any family history of suicide in family or close friends should be sought.

In first-attempt patients and patients of age over 60, there might be underlying medical co-morbidity with psychological symptoms. It is therefore recommended to perform routine screening for common conditions, including a full blood count, ferritin, iron studies and vitamin B12, as anaemia may present with mood disorders and fatigue. Liver function tests are also useful to rule out liver damage that can result in inadequate clearance of drugs prescribed and illicit drugs that may affect cognitive function. Thyroid function should be assessed, as hyper- and hypothyroidism are common causes for altered moods.

There are several clinical scoring tools that can aid clinicians in managing such patients; one such tool is the SADPERSONS scale:

- **Sex** (Male) (1 point)
- **Age** (<19 or >45) (1 point)
- **D**epression/Hopelessness (2 points)
- **P**revious attempt/Psychiatric admission (1 point)
- **E**toh (alcohol)/drug abuse (1 point)
- **R**ational thinking loss (2 points)
- **S**eperated/Divorced/Single (1 point)
- **O**rganised or serious attempt (2 points)
- **N**o social support (1 point)
- **S**tated future attempt (2 points)

Scores of 0–5 can be considered for discharge if medically stable, with mental health follow-up (or as per local policy). Scores between 6 and 8 should warrant an urgent review by a mental health specialist, and a score of >8 indicates that the patient requires inpatient admission to a mental health unit.

Most Emergency Departments have mental health liaison teams available 24 hours who will provide assessments for patients presenting to the ED. For those that are discharged home after risk assessment, ensure they access to crisis lines via telephone and remind them that they can represent to the ED if they feel like they are not coping. Often, the acute MH presentation is a cry for help, and a few extra minutes of time spent with the patient can prove invaluable to prevent subsequent attempts.

Ensure that documentation of presentation, attempts, suicide notes (handwritten, emails, SMS messages), capacity assessments and other multi-disciplinary assessment are contemporaneous in case of representation or should the need arise to formally place the patient under mental health act 'section'.

Table 36.1 **Potential risk factors and protective factors**

Risk factor	Protective factors
• Unemployed or recent financial difficulties • Divorced, separated, widowed • Social isolation • Prior traumatic life events or abuse • Previous suicide behaviour • Chronic mental illness • Chronic, debilitating physical ilness	• Strong family relationships or community • Skills in problem solving and conflict resolution • Sense of belonging and self-worth • Cultural and spiritual beliefs • Future goals • Enjoys activities • Willingness to seek and receive help • Restricted access to highly lethal means of suicide

Table 36.2 **Red flags**

- Threatening to harm or end one's life
- Seeking or access to means to self-harm
- Expression of suicide plan
- Writing or talking about suicide
- Hopelessness, helpless or feels trapped with no way out
- Rage or revenge-seeking behaviour
- Engaging in impulsive behaviour
- Anxiety and/or disturbed sleep
- Labile mood

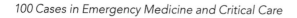 Key Points
• Self-harm is a complex behaviour that is not intended to end life. • Self-harm is associated with 100-fold increase risk of suicide, which represents a public health concern. • Males under 19 or over 45 years of age are more like to be successful in committing suicide often with severe acts.

NEUROLOGY AND NEUROSURGERY

CASE 37: BACK PAIN AT THE GYM

History

A 45-year-old man presents with acute onset lower back pain after a gym session. He limps into the Emergency Department several hours later and complains of weakness in his lower extremities, which came on with the back pain. He also has some pain and numbness down his legs and on the top of his feet, right worse than left. The pain has not been relieved by ibuprofen.

Examination

He is unable to walk on his heels. His abdomen is soft, but he has a large palpable mass below the umbilicus. A rectal exam reveals no active or passive tone.

| Investigations
| • An MRI of the lumbar spine is shown in Figure 37.1.

Questions

1. What is the diagnosis?
2. What imaging study/studies would you obtain?
3. Where would you expect to find the abnormality/abnormalities?
4. What else would you do?

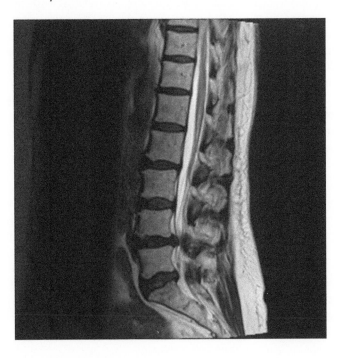

Figure 37.1 A sagittal section MRI scan of the lumbar spine.

DISCUSSION

This is a case of cauda equina syndrome (CES). The signs and symptoms of lower extremity weakness and pain developing acutely after heavy lifting should raise suspicion for a herniated intervertebral disc, which is the commonest cause of CES. Depending on the location and degree of the herniation, a combination of nerve root and cord could be impinged. In this case, the patient's foot drop and numbness in the anterior leg and dorsum of the feet suggest that the herniated disc was causing an L5 radiculopathy. The spinal cord typically terminates at the L1/2 level in an adult. Caudal to this, the cord continues as the cauda equina. If the spinal cord itself is compressed by a herniated disc, myelopathic signs such as hyperreflexia, Hoffmann's sign, Babinski's sign and clonus would be expected.

When the cauda equina is compressed by a very large central disc, patients can present with a combination of urinary retention, bowel incontinence, loss of anal tone and saddle anaesthesia. These findings are related to the compression of the somatic and autonomic fibres from nerve roots S2–4, which control the detrussor muscle of the bladder, external and internal anal sphincters and perineal sensation. The caliber of the spinal canal can also be reduced by osteophytes and soft tissue such as ligamentum flavum hypertrophy. In these cases, a smaller degree of herniated nucleus pulposus will produce marked signs and symptoms.

CES is a neurosurgical emergency. The goal is to prevent irreversible loss of bowel and bladder function and motor function of the lower extremities. While CES is primarily a clinical diagnosis, further imaging will be required to aid decision-making and operative planning. Ultimately, an MRI of the lumbar spine will help guide the neurosurgeon. In this case, the large L4/5 disc is seen to compress the cauda equina at this level with loss of CSF signal surrounding the nerve roots. Sagittal and axial T2 sequence images should be inspected to make this determination. Reproducible examination findings correlating with imaging findings strengthens the case for CES. A rectal exam to assess passive and active rectal tone as well as saddle anaesthesia is crucial; further, while urinary incontinence is erroneously thought of as a classic symptom, urinary retention remains the most common deficit associated with CES. A post-void bladder scan to assess residuals is a very helpful means of objectively diagnosing urinary retention. The timing of onset and duration of each symptom are particularly important to ascertain. A foot drop developing over the last 24 hours is more likely to improve with urgent decompression than bowel incontinence that has been ongoing for several weeks. Nevertheless, surgery may still be indicated in the latter case to prevent further deterioration in other aspects of the patient's neurological examination, especially if some function is still preserved.

A multitude of alternative diagnoses may masquerade as CES – stroke, vascular claudication, deep venous thrombosis, muscle cramps and peripheral neuropathy. A good history and examination will help differentiate these from true CES. If there is a concern for bony fracture from trauma, a non-contrast CT should be performed. If an unstable fracture is found on initial CT, spinal precautions should be maintained until definitive management. The scan time is in the order of seconds to minutes and hence will be available for inspection much quicker than an MRI, which can take 30–60 minutes. The lumbar spine is often scanned in isolation, but consideration should be given to extending the imaging to the thoracic and cervical spine as well as the brain in order to rule out a higher level lesion in cases where clinical correlation is less than expected.

While awaiting an MRI, a full blood count, electrolytes, coagulation studies and a group and save should be obtained in anticipation of surgical intervention. Obtained early, any pertinent abnormalities can be corrected with minimal delay in getting the patient into the operating theatre.

 Key Points

- Obtain a good history to rule out other pathology and always perform a rectal exam if cauda equine syndrome is suspected.
- Consider scanning the thoracic and cervical spine and/or the brain to rule out a higher lesion where indicated.
- Always compare with previous imaging if available.

History

A 17-year-old male student is brought to the Emergency Department after being punched from the side in a boxing match. He passed out but quickly regained consciousness. He complains of a throbbing headache and nausea, and has also vomited twice.

Examination

Screening cervical spine, central and peripheral nerve exams are normal. Abbreviated mental test score is 9/10.

Questions

1. Would you order a CT scan of the head? Justify your answer.
2. What other aspects of his history are important to explore?
3. What advice would you give the patient and his parents?

DISCUSSION

The basic principles of Advanced Trauma Life Support should be applied when dealing with this patient. Major injuries to rule out include cervical spine fractures or ligamentous injuries, intracranial bleeding and blunt cerebrovascular injuries. Imaging studies are not necessary in all cases, but should be considered if the clinical suspicion is high. The NICE guidelines on head injury state that a CT scan is indicated if any of the following are present:

- GCS < 13 on initial assessment
- GCS < 15 at 2 hours after injury on assessment in the Emergency Department
- Suspected open or depressed skull fracture
- Any sign of basal skull fracture
- Post-traumatic seizure
- Focal neurological deficit
- More than one episode of vomiting since the head injury
- Dangerous mechanism of injury
- Anti-coagulant use (e.g. warfarin, NOACs)
- >30 minutes of retrograde amnesia

In this case, as the patient has vomited twice post head injury, a non-contrast CT scan of the head would be indicated to rule out skull fracture and/or subdural haematoma with the lateral head injury. The CT scan in this case is normal.

Concussion is typically managed in the outpatient setting. While the most important aspects of the ED encounter include ruling out life- and limb-threatening injuries, establishing a diagnosis of concussion can have profound impact on the long-term outcomes of the individual. A suspicion of concussion should prompt a referral to a concussion expert. Depending on local practice, this could be a General Practitioner with an interest in sports medicine, a neurologist or a neurosurgeon. In larger centres, these specialists often work together in the evaluation and management of the patient.

The patient should be advised to avoid contact or collision sports until further evaluation and clearance by a concussion specialist. Young athletes in particular should not be allowed to return to play due to the risk of Second Impact Syndrome. In the acute period after a concussion, the patient is particularly vulnerable to further injury as a result of impaired reaction and decision-making abilities.

One of the key elements to establish is the concussion history of the patient. A history of multiple concussions, each with progressively longer recovery times, should prompt warning to the patient that further injury could lead to substantially greater morbidity and mortality. The effects of performance-enhancing drugs and illicit substance use in a concussed individual are controversial but should be taken into account, and screening should be considered. The use of helmets, while protective to a certain extent, does little to prevent rotational injuries.

No treatment has been proven to speed recovery from a concussion. Some advocate for strict rest (no physical activities, no reading, no television/computers/phones) for 5–7 days, but compliance will be an issue. Others have suggested an early active rehabilitation approach including strict rest in the first day or two, followed by the gradual introduction of mental activities and subsequently progressively intense physical activities.

In this case, with a negative CT scan, the patient should be discharged, provided there is someone on hand to supervise him at home, with both written and verbal instructions of the normal symptoms of concussion and red flags such as increased drowsiness, seizures, focal neurology and ongoing vomiting. Should the patient deteriorate at home or if the carer is concerned, they should return to the ED for reassessment. On occasion, patients may have delayed bleeds, which may necessitate re-scanning.

> **Key Points**
>
> - Rule out life- and limb-threatening injuries when dealing with a suspected concussion injury.
> - Establish a diagnosis of concussion based on high clinical suspicion.
> - Refer the patient to a concussion specialist for further outpatient evaluation and management.
> - Always discharge patients with head injury into the care of a relative with both verbal and written head injury instructions detailing normal concussive symptoms and when to return to the ED.

History

A 45-year-old female presents to the Emergency Department with confusion. She is not following commands but can localise to pain. According to her partner, she was complaining of a severe headache when she started vomiting and became less coherent in her speech.

Examination

She is unable to tolerate light being shined into her eyes. Her right pupil is larger than her left and is not reactive to light. She has a right adduction gaze palsy.

 Investigations
- A non-contrast CT brain is obtained (Figure 39.1).

Questions

1. Describe the findings on the CT scan. What is the likely underlying cause?
2. Is a lumbar puncture indicated?
3. What other investigations would you perform in the ED?
4. How would you manage this patient?

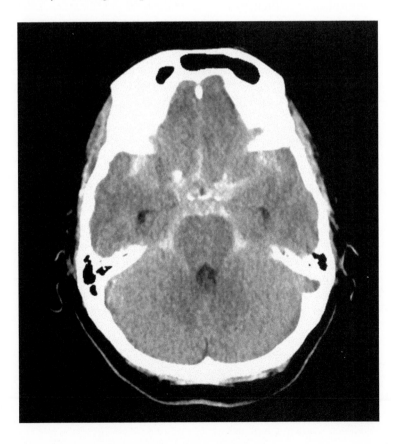

Figure 39.1 A non-contrast axial section CT of the brain.

DISCUSSION

The non-contrast CT brain shows hyperdensity in the basal cisterns extending into the sylvian fissure and posteriorly into the ambient cisterns, consistent with subarachnoid haemorrhage (SAH). This classic star-shaped appearance of SAH raises concern for a ruptured aneurysm. Given this patient's right third nerve involvement (loss of parasympathetic innervation leading to pupillary dilatation, loss of motor function leading to adduction palsy), a posterior cerebral artery or posterior communicating artery aneurysm on the right would be the most likely cause.

Given that a diagnosis of SAH has been obtained, there is little additional value in performing a lumbar puncture (LP). In cases where SAH is suspected but a CT head does not show evidence of a bleed, an LP with three serial samples performed to look for red blood cell count and xanthochromia is most sensitive between 12 and 24 hours of ictus. A non-contrast CT is most sensitive close to the onset of ictus, with sensitivity decreasing with time due to clot resolution. The hyperdensity seen is due to the high density of stagnant haemoglobin, which contains iron.

After a diagnosis of SAH is obtained, the next step in consultation with neurosurgery would be to identify the source of the SAH and other unrupted aneurysms or arteriovenous malformations (AVMs). An initial, quick, increasingly sensitive and non-invasive modality of achieving this is through a CT angiogram (CTA) of the head. A CTA also has the additional benefit of identifying contrast blush or extravasation, which would point to the source of rupture. This may supersede the need for an LP, which is a more invasive procedure. An MRI/MR angiogram is occasionally necessary but is less sensitive for small or thrombosed aneurysms. The current gold standard is a catheter digital subtraction angiogram of the cerebral vasculature. While this is invasive and not typically performed in the acute setting, it has the benefit of enabling concurrent endovascular treatment of the ruptured aneurysm.

A proportion of patients with ruptured aneurysms do not make it in time to the ED. Those that do make it usually have a clot tamponading the focus of rupture. The risk of re-rupture in the acute period is high, and blood pressure should be controlled as soon as possible. Typically, IV hydralazine or labetalol is administered, depending on the patient's heart rate, to keep the systolic pressures below 140–160. A nimodipine infusion may be necessary. However, depending on the patient's baseline blood pressure, caution is advised against dropping it more than 20% in the acute phase.

Another common early sequela of SAH is hydrocephalus, especially in the setting of intraventricular haemorrhage, causing CSF outflow/resorption obstruction. These patients will require an external ventricular drain (EVD) to relieve the CSF build-up. Neurosurgery should be consulted as soon as a CT brain is available demonstrating SAH. If not already done prior to this, a full set of blood tests including coagulation panel should be sent in anticipation of imminent intervention.

 | Key Points

- A CT head should be performed urgently in all cases where intracranial haemorrhage is suspected.
- In cases of SAH, the initial focus is to control blood pressure, aiming to maintain systolic <140–160, due to a high risk of re-rupture.
- Patients need to be observed closely to monitor for development of hydrocephalus.

History

A 35-year-old man is the unrestrained driver in a head-on motor vehicle accident. At the scene, he was found to be unresponsive. Paramedics intubated him and rushed him to the Emergency Department.

Examination

On arrival, he has clear breath sounds bilaterally. His pulse is 110 and his blood pressure is 170/90 mm Hg. He twitches to pinching of his limbs, but does not open his eyes or make any verbal sounds. His left pupil is 6 mm and sluggish; his right pupil is 3 mm and briskly reactive. Apart from some facial lacerations, lacerations and abrasions on his forearms, he has no other obvious external injuries.

 Investigations
  • A CT scan of the head is shown in Figure 40.1.

Questions

1. What is the patient's Glasgow Coma Scale (GCS) score?
2. What is the diagnosis? What are your other differentials and how do you differentiate between them?
3. What are the next steps in managing this patient?

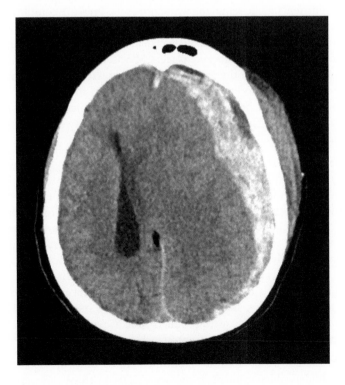

Figure 40.1 A non-contrast axial section CT of the brain.

DISCUSSION

This is a common presentation in head trauma patients. The basic principles of Advanced Trauma Life Support (ATLS) should be followed – Airway with cervical spine immobilisation, Breathing and Circulation, in that order, should take priority over obtaining the CT head. As a part of the primary survey, the patient's Glasgow Coma Scale (GCS) score is assessed by eliciting the best Eye (E), Verbal (V) and Motor (M) responses. In this example, the patient scores an E1 V1 M1 at the scene, and E1 V_T (intubated) M4 on arrival at the Trauma Centre. The GCS is an objective and reproducible clinical tool to classify the severity of brain injury and monitor for clinical deterioration and improvement. The motor component is important as it helps predict long-term neurological outcome.

In this case, the patient's CT scan of the head shows a hyperdense crescent-shaped area beneath the skull, causing mass effect on the underlying brain parenchyma. There is also midline shift and effacement of the lateral ventricle on the left. This is the classic appearance of an acute subdural haematoma (SDH). An acute SDH originates from venous bleeding, typically from dural bridging veins that sheer from the rapid acceleration–deceleration movements experienced by the brain from trauma. Depending on the extent of the injury and the amount of space in the cranial vault, the patient could remain neurologically stable or could deteriorate as evidenced by a drop in the GCS and development of a motor deficit.

Blood in the subdural space occupies the limited space inside the skull. In a normal individual, this space is filled primarily with brain matter. The brain is surrounded by cerebrospinal fluid (CSF), which acts as a shock absorber to protect the brain against the hard (and often rough) surface of the skull. Blood vessels travel into and out of the skull to supply the brain with oxygen and nutrients while removing waste products. Pressure equilibrium in the fixed cavity of the skull is maintained through the relationship of the volume of the brain matter, CSF and blood in the skull. With the introduction of an additional compartment, in the form of subdural blood, a number of events take place. CSF will be displaced out of the skull, and occasionally, the outflow tract of the CSF could be compressed by brain matter, leading to obstructive hydrocephalus. Blood vessels are compressed and therefore blood supply to the brain is compromised. Finally, brain matter may herniate, manifesting as dilated pupils and eventually respiratory arrest. This finely balanced relationship between the intracranial compartments is known as the Monro–Kellie doctrine.

The goal in these scenarios is to prevent secondary brain injury. Injury from the initial trauma (primary brain injury) may have caused irreversible damage to some brain tissue. Secondary brain injury can be prevented through prompt evaluation and treatment of trauma patients. Once a diagnosis is confirmed through a non-contrast head CT, neurosurgical consultation should be obtained. Depending on the local practice patterns, the neurosurgeon may or may not be a part of the initial trauma team evaluating the patient on arrival. The decision to take the patient to surgery for decompression is not straightforward and is often based on clinical judgement and radiological findings. Several factors could be optimised in the early phases of the patient's encounter. These include early blood tests, including a full blood count, coagulation labs and a group and save in anticipation of operative interventions. Obtained early, this will enable time for correction with products such as packed red blood cells, platelets, vitamin K and prothrombin complex concentrate where indicated.

Occasionally, the patient either does not require emergent surgical decompression or is a poor surgical candidate. Management of the acute SDH in these instances should follow the basic principles of intracranial pressure (ICP) management. First tier strategies, such as raising the head of the bed or adopting a reverse Trendelenburg position for patients with concomitant spinal injuries, ensuring unobstructed venous jugular outflow and maintaining normothermia, should be employed initially. If indicated, an ICP monitor should be placed to help guide resuscitation. At this point, patients will typically have a GCS < 8 and would require intubation.

Cerebral oedema can be reduced by driving interstitial fluid into the cerebrovascular circulation and eventually out of the 'fixed box'. Agents commonly employed include hypertonic saline and mannitol. An intubated and ventilated patient comes with the benefit of being able to control the pCO_2 level through the ventilator to induce cerebro-vasoconstriction. Due to the risk of inadequate perfusion, this technique is controversial and should only be used sparingly. Sedation and muscle paralytics can lower the metabolic demands of the body and hence increase oxygen delivery to the brain. Hypothermia, which should theoretically achieve similar goals, has been controversial and should be avoided due to the risk of coagulopathy. CSF diversion is often performed via the insertion of an external ventricular drain (EVD), which carries the additional benefit of enabling ICP monitoring.

 Key Points

- Always adhere to ATLS principles when assessing patients with head injury.
- Obtain a non-contrast CT head as soon as feasible when a subdural haemorrhage is suspected.
- Intubate the patient if necessary, but obtain a good examination beforehand and use short-acting and reversible medications to enable repeat examinations to guide interventions.
- Remember that time is brain.

History

A 63-year-old man is brought into the Emergency Department after crashing into the car in front while driving on a quiet street. His wife noticed his speech began to slur immediately prior to the crash. He has a history of hypertension, controlled on amlodipine and hydro-chlorothiazide, and hyperlipidemia, for which he takes a statin. He is a current smoker of 30 pack years.

Examination

Vital signs: temperature of 36.8°C, blood pressure of 180/90, heart rate of 80 and regular, respiratory rate of 18, 96% O$_2$ saturation on air.

He is unable to fully support himself while standing and his left arm is shaking as he grips the railing for support. The right arm appears limp. Pin-prick sensation and reflexes on the right are diminished, with the upper extremity worse than the lower extremity. His visual fields are grossly intact.

Questions

1. What is the diagnosis?
2. What are the principles of workup and management of this patient?
3. What investigations would you prioritise?

DISCUSSION

This is a trauma situation, and not infrequently, such events are precipitated by a medical condition, like a myocardial infarction, seizure or, as in this case, a stroke. Depending on local practices, the mechanism of injury and severity of injuries from the initial triage assessment, a trauma call may have been activated from the pre-hospital setting.

Once the primary survey has taken place and the patient does not require any further lifesaving interventions from a trauma standpoint, a focused and thorough history from the patient and any family member present is warranted if the suspicion of a precipitating event like a stroke is high. Key items to establish are the time of onset or time known well, history of any previous strokes, premorbid functional status, use of anticoagulants and an assessment of the patient's National Institutes of Health Stroke Score (NIHSS) at presentation. The NIHSS is a 15-part neurologic examination that evaluates the severity of a possible stroke by assessing various brain functions, including consciousness, speech, language, neglect, vision, eye movements and motor and sensory function. It should be performed in *all* patients with a suspected stroke, and it ordinarily takes only a few minutes; in addition to assessing the severity, it can be used to monitor neurologic improvement.

Going down the stroke pathway, further evaluation and treatment should be based on the understanding that the damage that is done (infarcted brain) is likely to be permanent, and the goal is to prevent further damage (ischaemic brain) and treat reversible causes (secondary prevention). Along those lines, time is critical to the outcome of the patient. Depending on local practice, protocols exist for stroke activation, which should be initiated as early as possible. Further workup will then take place in conjunction with a stroke physician, but nevertheless, the ED physician should be familiar with the basic concepts. One of the initial key steps would be determining the type of stroke – ischaemic versus haemorrhagic – with an emergent non-contrast CT head, as management is fundamentally different.

In patients with ischaemic stroke, reperfusion therapy (thrombolysis and mechanical thrombectomy) has evolved into a larger role in management, in an attempt to salvage ischaemic but not infarcted brain. Intravenous tPA (alteplase) has been shown to improve functional independence and reduce mortality in selected patients (ischaemic stroke patients within 4.5 hours of onset or last known well) without contraindications (haemorrhagic conversion, large area of infarcted brain, recent stroke/myocardial infarction, coagulopathy).

Over the past 5 years, several trials have demonstrated a benefit in the use of mechanical thrombectomy, particularly for large vessel occlusion of the anterior circulation. A CT angiogram of the head and neck will be required, ideally performed at the same time as the CT head to minimise unnecessary transport and delays. As with tPA, mechanical thrombectomy has risks, with similar contraindications to that associated with tPA. In centres without stroke interventionalists, a treat and transfer model may be adopted if the patient has a reasonable chance of achieving groin puncture by 6 hours of symptom onset or last known well.

Blood tests usually will be available within 30 minutes and should be initiated early on regardless of the diagnosis. Besides coagulation studies, serum glucose and cardiac enzymes should be performed to rule out stroke mimics such as hypoglycaemia and myocardial infarction, respectively. It also enables correction of hyperglycaemia, which has been shown to be associated with poor outcomes in acute stroke (higher risk of haemorrhagic conversion in reperfusion therapy, worse ischaemic damage). An accurate body weight should be obtained as this will enable accurate dosing of tPA.

Once the acute evaluation is performed to enable a decision to be made regarding reperfusion therapy, further workup is then aimed at secondary prevention.

 Key Points

- Stroke is a medical emergency; any patient with a suspected stroke requires a neurologic examination to calculate the NIHSS.
- A CT head is emergently needed in suspected stroke to look for haemorrhage.
- Always establish the timing of symptom onset or when the patient was last known to be well, as thrombolysis is typically only performed for patients presenting within 4.5 hours of symptom onset.

History

A 50-year-old male presents with confusion. He localises on the right more briskly than the left. He is able to speak but he does not seem to make much sense. The left side of his face is less animated compared to the right. He chokes on a sip of water in the Emergency Department. His son reports that he had been normal until a sudden change while cooking, resulting in a fall with him landing face first.

Examination

Vital signs: temperature of 36.8°C, heart rate of 90, blood pressure of 200/130, respiratory rate of 18, 95% O_2 saturation on air.

He has a small laceration on his lip and mild periorbital swelling on the left. He is unable to open his left eye, but his pupils are equal and reactive. When asked to raise his arms up in the air, he is only able to lift his right arm, with which he demonstrated good hand–eye coordination. He indicates numbness on the left side of his body, and reflexes are less brisk on the left compared to the right.

Investigations
• A CT scan of the brain is shown in Figure 42.1.

Questions

1. What are the likely diagnoses?
2. What are the principles of workup and management of this patient?

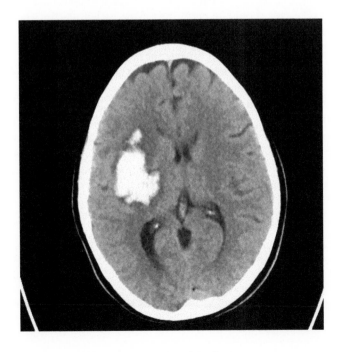

FIGURE 42.1   A non-contrast axial section CT of the brain.

DISCUSSION

This is a case of a stroke. The initial assessment and management is similar to that of the previous case ('slurred speech and weakness'). The patient should be stabilised from an 'ABCDE' standpoint, and a CT brain scan should be obtained as soon as possible. Stroke mimics should also be ruled out along the way, but this should not impede a stroke workup.

The CT brain scan shows a hyperdense mass lesion in the right putamen, a classic finding of a hypertensive stroke. It is often difficult to differentiate this from a haemorrhagic conversion of an ischaemic stroke. However, given that this will mean that reperfusion therapy will be contraindicated, further workup and management at this point should be directed towards that of a haemorrhagic stroke. Common causes of haemorrhagic stroke include hypertension and cerebral amyloid angiopathy. Vascular anomalies like arteriovenous malformations (AVMs) and cavernomas should be ruled out with an MRI or MR angiography in due course.

One of the earliest interventions that should be initiated is strict blood pressure control. This is to minimise the risk of rebleeding. Typically, IV hydralazine or labetalol is administered, depending on the patient's heart rate, to keep the systolic pressure below 140–160 mmHg. However, depending on the patient's baseline blood pressure, caution is advised against reducing the systolic pressure by more than 20% in the acute phase. Other simple measures for intracranial pressure management should be considered (see case on 'motor vehicle accident' for further discussion).

A full set of blood tests should be obtained including a coagulation panel. Any coagulopathy should be corrected, with anticoagulants withheld, due to the risk of haematoma expansion. There is a high risk of haematoma expansion in the first 6–12 hours even in a non-coagulopathic patient. These patients will need an admission to the High Dependency Unit. Close monitoring and frequent examinations are important to detect a decline in neurological status. Repeat CT scans should be performed if the patient declines neurologically, but also at intervals determined by local practice.

Surgical evacuation of intracranial haemorrhage has been studied previously without strong evidence showing benefit over medically managed patients in terms of mortality and functional outcome. Nevertheless, Neurosurgery should be consulted early on, along with the stroke team, due to the possibility of hydrocephalus (especially in the event of the haematoma extending into the ventricles) requiring an external ventricular drain (EVD) or the need for a decompressive craniectomy. Several trials are ongoing to investigate the utility of a minimally invasive approach to surgically evacuate the haematoma. Cerebellar haemorrhage may require emergent decompression due to the lack of room for mass expansion. Steroids are not particularly useful in reducing oedema in this setting.

Key Points
• Common causes for a hypertensive stroke include poorly controlled hypertension and cerebral amyloid angiopathy.
• Control systolic blood pressures to 140–160 mm Hg in such cases, but take care not to reduce the pressure by more than 20% acutely.
• A CT or MR angiogram is needed in such cases to rule out vascular malformations that could be intervened upon.
• EVD or decompressive craniectomy may be required to relieve hydrocephalus.

History

A 74-year-old woman with a history of type 2 diabetes presents to the Emergency Department after a road traffic accident. She reports neck pain, numbness in her hands bilaterally and urinary incontinence.

Examination

Her upper extremities are symmetrically weak. Her right lower extremity is slightly weaker than the left, and she complains of hip pain that is worse with movement. Reflexes are normal and she has extensor Babinski responses blaterally.

 | Investigations

• A sagittal slice of a CT scan of the cervical spine is shown in Figure 43.1.

Questions

1. What are the priorities in this patient's management?
2. What are the key aspects in evaluating this patient?
3. What type of imaging is shown and what are the pertinent findings?

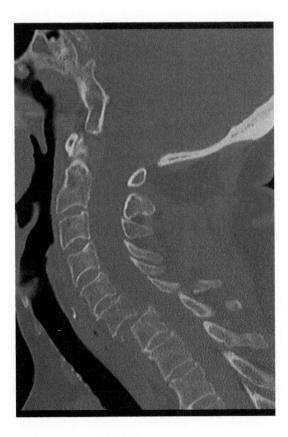

Figure 43.1   A sagittal slice of CT cervical spine.

DISCUSSION

In any patient where trauma is involved, management should proceed in accordance with Advanced Trauma Life Support (ATLS) guidelines. Many of these patients will arrive on a spinal board. As part of the secondary survey, the patient should be log-rolled onto a standard bed. It is often not possible to clear the patient's spine in the acute phase especially when other issues take precedence. When in doubt, the patient should always be placed on strict full spine precautions until sufficient clinical and/or radiographic evidence is available to enable spinal clearance. When clearing the patient clinically, an accurate assessment of neck pain and focal motor deficits with passive and active range of movements will need to be demonstrated. For this, the patient will need to be free from any potential distractors and confounders (pain elsewhere, intoxication, cognitive impairment).

When performing the primary survey, it is important to consider a high spinal cord injury as a potential cause for any breathing difficulties. If a spine injury is suspected, a CT scan should be obtained of the appropriate level. If in doubt, it would not be unreasonable to scan the whole spine. Depending on local imaging protocols, if a CT scan of the chest, abdomen or pelvis is obtained, the thoracic and lumbar spine sequences can often be reconstructed from the former.

In this case, the image shows a distraction injury of C6/7. This is an unstable injury and has caused narrowing of the spinal canal. A comprehensive neurologic exam should be documented as soon as possible after presentation. This will serve to guide the timing of further intervention, and as a baseline for comparison after future interventions. This patient will need a reduction of her dislocated cervical spine. Disruption of the ligaments has the potential to cause an epidural haematoma, which may not be obviously seen on a CT scan. In a patient where a clinical exam is possible, it is prudent to perform serial examinations to monitor for any potential epidural haematoma causing cord compression. MRI may delineate the injury more clearly and this may need urgent surgical decompression.

While a clinical examination is sensitive for new changes, its specificity suffers from other disease processes masquerading as a spine problem. This lady has diabetes, which could cause peripheral neuropathy and explain her hand numbness. Her gait instability and urinary incontinence could suggest a myelopathy further down in the thoracic or lumbar spine. Lower extremity pain could be explained by claudication or osteoarthritis. The latter is most likely in her case, but in the setting of a trauma, a hip or pelvic fracture will need to be ruled out. In the elderly, these alternative diagnoses should be explored and ruled out as appropriate.

 Key Points

- In a trauma situation, always ensure spinal precautions are observed until the spine can be 'cleared' either clinically or radiologically.
- Remember that C3, 4, 5 keep the diaphragm alive.
- Always perform a thorough neurologic examination in patients presenting with possible spinal pathology, as this guides further evaluation and serves as a baseline for future comparison.

TRAUMA AND ORTHOPAEDICS

CASE 44: MY BACK HURTS

History

A 45-year-old man who works in a retail outlet presents to the Urgent Treatment Centre with increasing lower back pain for the last 3–4 months. His job involves administration and he occasionally has to restock shelves due to staff shortages. Of late, the pain is worse at the end of the day and sometimes radiates down his left leg. He has required some time off work, and his General Practitioner has tried giving simple ibuprofen but he finds that this is not helping anymore. The patient is demanding an x-ray of his back.

Examination

Peripheral neurological examination demonstrates normal tone in both legs, power 5/5 on the MRC scale at the hip, knee, ankle, foot and toes. There is no objective reduction in sensation in either leg or the perineum and normal peripheral reflexes. Active straight leg raising is 90 degrees on the right but only 60 degrees on the left side, limited by pain. The sciatic stretch test is positive on the left. The patient's gait is antalgic with a pronounced limp.

Questions

1. What is the diagnosis and initial management?
2. How would you respond to his request for a plain radiograph of his spine?
3. What would you tell him about prognosis and return to work?

DISCUSSION

This man is suffering from mechanical back pain. Mechanical back pain is the term given to back pain which is of a structural cause. This may originate from anywhere from the paraspinal muscles, vertebral joints or intervertebral discs and is primarily caused by a physical problem.

In this case, the patient is suffering from sciatica as indicated by pain radiating down the left leg. The sciatic nerve originates from the lumbosacral plexus from the roots of L4-S3. It passes down from the gluteal region into the posterior compartment of the thigh where it supplies the hamstring muscles and adductor magnus, and then into the calf via the popliteal fossa to supply the calf, the whole of the lower leg and muscles of the foot. The sensory distribution therefore is classically the posterior thigh, lower leg and the foot.

Sciatica is primarily a physical problem whereby lumbar intervertebral discs become dehydrated usually with age and use and then prolapse causing impingement of exiting nerve roots. The extent of symptoms depends on the number of discs involved, the degree of prolapse and direction – left, right or centrally, which is much worse prognostically (typified by 'bilateral' sciatica, a red flag sign).

In this case, the diagnosis was confirmed with a positive sciatic stretch test. Assessment of these patients requires careful neurological evaluation including the perineum to exclude saddle anaesthesia and assessment of anal sphincter tone and bladder volume to exclude cauda equina syndrome.

Management of patients with mechanical back pain is stepwise. You should start with education on why this pain occurs and the underlying cause with education on proper lifting techniques and posture. Formal physiotherapy can prove to be vital in this aspect.

In terms of drug therapy for pain, current guidance is to follow the World Health Organization pain ladder with paracetamol, NSAIDs in the lowest effective dose with consideration of gastro-protection and a weak opioid. In the acute setting, low-dose diazepam may be considered for a few days if there is a significant component of spasm.

With neuropathic pain such as sciatica, amitriptyline or gabapentin may be offered, but this requires careful monitoring and dose titration and may be more suited to prescription via his GP or a specialist pain clinic.

Some patients may ask about other therapies such as corsets, back braces, TENS machines, 'spinal ultrasound' and 'spinal manipulations'. These are currently not recommended as the evidence base for their efficacy is poor. Acupuncture was previously recommended for some patients but has been removed from the current NICE guidelines.

In terms of imaging, plain radiographs are not recommended with mechanical back pain or sciatica. Due to the underlying cause (i.e. disc, facet joint or paraspinal muscular problems), they are often normal and result in unnecessary radiation exposure. However, if you suspect fracture or lytic/sclerotic bone lesions, they may have some diagnostic yield. The imaging modality of choice is MRI, and this is normally arranged via a specialist spinal clinic or via an urgent outpatient basis in cases of prolonged pain or radiculopathy.

Most episodes of back pain resolve in 6 weeks with mobilisation and anti-inflammatory therapy, but 1 in 10 episodes last longer. These patients should be referred to the local back pain service for multimodal assessment. Treatment depends on underlying cause, and a range of options are available, including supervised physiotherapy, caudal epidural injection and surgery.

His local work occupational health department should be involved as they can support him in his daily managerial role and may be able to provide reduced work hours, assessment of his seating area and limitation of heavy lifting as well as support for ongoing or recurrent flares.

 Key Points

- Mechanical back pain is very common.
- Assessment should include a detailed and thorough peripheral neurological examination to exclude cauda equina syndrome which is a neurosurgical emergency.
- Management should follow a stepwise approach of education, pharmacotherapy and mobilisation.
- Those with ongoing or prolonged symptoms should be referred to a specialist clinic for assessment and management.

CASE 45: MY SHOULDER POPPED OUT

History

A 21-year-old man was playing basketball at his local court. He approached a 'lay-up' shot and suddenly felt his shoulder give. He states that there is now a visible deformity and he cannot raise his arm. He arrived at the Emergency Department with his friend, bent over, holding the injured right arm flexed at the elbow and supported with his left hand. A first aider at the sports complex has applied a broad arm sling.

Examination

There is a visible deformity of the right shoulder with a squared off appearance compared to the other side. You assess his median, radial and ulnar nerve function (motor and sensory), sensation over 'regimental badge' area and radial pulse. There is no deficit.

 Investigations
- AP and lateral radiographs of the right shoulder are performed (Figure 45.1a and b).

Questions

1. What is the diagnosis?
2. Are there any associated injuries that you need to look for?
3. How are you going to manage this injury?
4. What would you do if the patient could not move their hand and had a concurrent neurological injury?

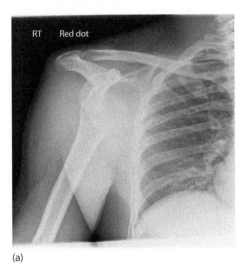

(a)

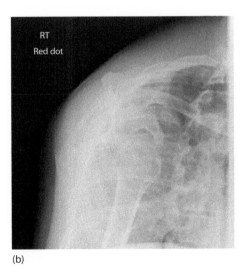

(b)

Figure 45.1 AP (a) and lateral (b) radiographs of the right shoulder.

DISCUSSION

This patient has an anterior dislocation of the shoulder. Dislocations of the glenohumeral (shoulder) joint occur when a large force is applied to the joint, tearing the stabilising joint capsule and the surrounding tissues. There are three types of dislocation – anterior, posterior and inferior – with the anterior type being most common. Radiographs are usually performed to confirm the diagnosis, but are not always required in recurrent cases.

Anterior dislocation is easily confirmed on the radiograph, but posterior dislocations are sometimes missed due to the subtle signs on anteroposterior (AP) projection – there is a characteristic 'light bulb' appearance of the humeral head. Inferior dislocations are rare but associated with epilepsy and trauma with an abducted arm. The patient typically presents with the arm fully abducted to 180 degrees and the elbow flexed – the 'tea-pot' position.

With shoulder dislocations, look for the following associated injuries:

1. *A fracture of the greater tuberosity.* This can be problematic as large fragments may obstruct relocation and it is the site of rotator cuff muscle attachment.
2. *The Bankart lesion.* This is a tear of the anterior inferior part of the labrum and sometimes a bony chip fragment may be visible on the radiograph.
3. *The Hill–Sachs lesion.* The posterior part of the humeral head may be fractured against the glenoid rim as the humeral head is dislocated. It is visible as a 'dent' in the humeral head on the radiograph.
4. *Neurological injuries.* The axillary nerve can be stretched and the patient may have altered sensation over the regimental badge area. This usually recovers on reduction. Occasionally there may be an associated brachial plexus injury and this should prompt immediate orthopaedic referral.

Management of simple anterior dislocation is usually straightforward. First, provide prompt analgesia (Entonox, oral or intravenous), perform a focused neurological exam and confirm the diagnosis radiographically. After that, a variety of techniques for reduction exist and these must be centred on patient choice, pain perception and the experience of the clinician. Most anterior dislocations, especially recurrent ones, can be reduced with only Entonox. Position the patient sitting upright with the shoulder slightly abducted and the elbow supported and flexed to 90 degrees. Gently externally rotate the humerus and the shoulder usually relocates. If the shoulder has not reduced with full external rotation, adduct elbow over the chest wall and internally rotate the arm to bring the wrist to lie on the opposite shoulder. This is referred to as Kocher's method. The key to all reductions is very slow movement and should the patient be in pain, to stop and wait. Gentle traction downwards also helps if the humeral head is wedged under the glenoid.

If the patient requires additional analgesia or chooses sedation, the patient must be moved to the resuscitation room, and a practitioner trained in sedation using appropriate monitoring must carry out the sedation whilst a second clinician carries out the reduction.

There are a number of other methods (e.g. traction only, scapular manipulation) for reduction and no single one has proved to be superior. Success is usually obtained with adequate analgesia, relaxation and an experienced operator.

Neurovascular checks should be carried out pre- and post-procedure and documented. The reduced shoulder should be immobilised in a collar and cuff sling or a poly-sling and a check radiograph performed. The patient should follow up in a fracture clinic for rehabilitation. Warn the patient not to fully abduct or externally rotate the arm as the shoulder may dislocate again.

If there is a pre-reduction neurological injury, an associated fracture or a failure of reduction in the emergency department, orthopaedic referral should be made promptly.

 Key Points

- Anterior dislocations are the most common type of shoulder dislocation.
- Assessment should include neurovascular checks pre- and post-reduction.
- The method of reduction should take into account pain, patient choice and the experience of the clinician.
- Orthopaedic referral is mandated in complex fracture dislocations and neurological injury.

History
A 65-year-old woman was returning home on the bus. As the bus was approaching the stop, a car pulled out in front causing the driver to brake suddenly. The woman was thrown forward and injured her arm against a metal handrail on the bus. She tells you that she has a lot of pain and she can feel something moving. A broad arm sling has been applied.

Examination
The left arm is very swollen compared to the other side and crepitus can be felt over the shaft of the humerus. Distal neurovascular function including the median, ulnar and radial nerves (motor and sensory) and the radial pulse are intact.

 Investigations
- AP and lateral radiographs of the left humerus are shown in Figures 46.1 and 46.2.

Questions
1. What is your initial management of the patient?
2. What potential complications should you look for?
3. How are you going to immobilise the fracture?

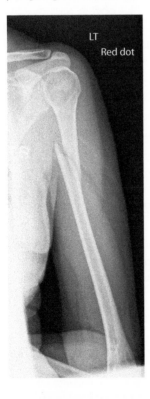
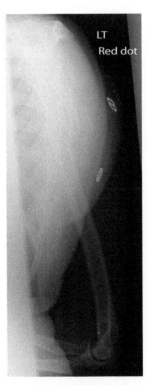

Figure 46.1 AP radiograph of the left humerus.

Figure 46.2 Lateral radiograph of the left humerus.

DISCUSSION

This lady has a spiral proximal humeral shaft fracture. This injury is associated with a rotational type injury such as holding a rail and being thrown forward. There can be significant soft tissue injury and internal bleeding, and so this should be assessed at the same time and documented. In addition, the radial nerve wraps around the middle portion of the humerus in the spiral groove and may be injured in up to 18% of midshaft fractures, and assessment should therefore document distal function.

The initial management of the patient should be along ATLS guidelines with a brief primary survey of the patient to exclude any other injuries including the cervical spine and then a focused exam of the arm, including the joint above and below.

Humeral shaft fractures tend to be very painful injuries and adequate analgesia should therefore be provided. Intravenous opioids may be required prior to imaging and will often improve the quality of radiographs. You should image the whole length of the humerus including the shoulder and elbow joints. There is no universally accepted classification system for humeral fractures, and a descriptive approach is best when communicating with orthopaedic surgeons. Management of these fractures follows the standard orthopaedic principles of 'reduce, hold and rehabilitate', and the majority of these fractures are treated conservatively.

A 'U-slab' cast extending in a sugar tong fashion along the humeral shaft length may be used to stabilise the fracture. A humeral brace may also be used as an alternative and is often tolerated well in younger patients with simple fractures. The alternative is a 'hanging cast', which is a plaster cast applied along the forearm including above the elbow that is flexed at 90 degrees and extends onto the humerus. The wrist is supported with a collar and cuff. The aim of this cast is to provide traction weight to overcome the contraction of the biceps and triceps.

Whichever method of immobilisation is chosen, adequate analgesia should be given to the patient and procedural sedation by a trained clinician is very useful. Radiographs should be taken post-procedure to check the reduction.

With certain fracture patterns and younger patients, operative fixation may be considered either by open reduction and internal fixation or intramedullary nail devices. Management may vary according to centres, and early advice from an upper limb orthopaedic surgeon is advised.

The older patient may need a period of observation in the Emergency Department prior to discharge. Often the injuries are to the dominant arm and cause significant morbidity even if being managed conservatively. Multidisciplinary assessment by physiotherapy and occupational therapists is invaluable.

 Key Points

- Humeral fractures may be associated with other injuries – always assess the patient according to ATLS principles.
- Assessment of the injury should encompass the soft tissue compartments and distal neurovascular status, in particular the radial nerve, which runs through the spiral groove.
- Seek early advice from orthopaedic specialists regarding operative versus conservative management.

CASE 47: MOTORBIKE RTC

History

A 45-year-old man is brought in to the Emergency Department resuscitation room as a trauma call. He came off his motorbike at around 10 mph in icy conditions. He laid the bike down onto the left-hand side and landed directly onto his elbow. On scene, he removed his helmet, sat up and walked to the pavement. He was wearing full armored riding gear and boots. His elbow is obviously deformed and the paramedics have applied a splint.

Examination

You examine him according to ATLS guidelines and the primary survey is unremarkable. The left elbow is obviously deformed and swollen. There is a small abrasion to the overlying skin but no obvious bone protrusion. Distal median, ulnar and radial nerve function is normal. However, his hand is cool and mottled, with a capillary refill time of more than 2 seconds.

 Investigations

- Radiographs of the elbow show a multi-fragmentary supracondylar elbow fracture.

Questions

1. What is your initial management of this fracture?
2. What structure has potentially been damaged?
3. How are you going to immobilise this fracture?

DISCUSSION

This man has a complex supracondylar fracture of the humerus with vascular compromise.

Supracondylar fractures in the adult are relatively uncommon but are seen in major trauma or in elderly patients where bone quality may be compromised. Elbow fractures need careful neurovascular evaluation as well as examination of shoulder and wrist joints.

There are three major nerves that pass through the region:

1. The median nerve enters the elbow joint anterior and medial to the brachial artery and then descends to give branches to the anterior (flexor) compartment of the forearm. It also gives rise to the anterior interosseous nerve (AIN), which runs along the interosseous membrane. The median nerve or AIN branch is most commonly injured in elbow fractures.
2. The radial nerve winds around the humerus in the spiral groove and enters the elbow anterior to the lateral epicondyle to supply the posterior (extensor) compartment of the forearm.
3. The ulnar nerve travels posteromedially at the elbow joint and then enters the forearm giving branches the flexor carpi ulnaris and the medial half of the flexor digitorum profundus before supplying the intrinsic muscles of the hand and the thumb.

It is important to assess these three nerves and to document their function individually. A quick method of doing this is to ask the patient to perform the hand actions to the game 'rock, paper, scissors'. The individual hand positions provide a quick assessment of individual nerve function as follows: rock – median nerve, paper – radial nerve and posterior interosseous nerve, scissors – ulnar nerve and the 'ok' sign – anterior interosseous nerve.

The brachial artery passes through the cubital fossa and may be directly injured by bone fragments or suffer intimal damage. In this case, the patient has a cool and mottled hand, which strongly suggests a vascular injury. You should try and palpate the distal wrist pulses and call for immediate vascular and orthopaedic help. In the Emergency Department, gently flexing or extending the elbow by as little as 15 degrees may result in reperfusion of the hand. A temporary above elbow plaster backslab should be applied in this position. The forearm compartments should also be assessed for compartment syndrome prior to application of plaster.

The patient will need to be transferred to theatre for open reduction and internal fixation of the fracture and repair of any vascular structures. This is a true orthopaedic and vascular emergency as the upper limb can only tolerate an ischaemia time of around 90 minutes before irreparable damage is sustained. A dual approach by orthopaedic and vascular surgeons is normally required.

 Key Points

- Adult supracondylar fractures are associated with high kinetic energy injuries.
- Carefully document neurovascular status in all cases down to the individual nerve and artery.
- Most of these injuries are treated with operative fixation and will need referral to the orthopaedic team.

History

A 55-year-old woman was walking to the train station in wet weather. The steps down to the platform were wet and she slipped on the last step to the platform. She broke her fall with her outstretched hand. At the train station, one of the staff applied a broad arm sling and the patient called a taxi to the hospital. The triage nurse assessed her pain score on arrival and has provided paracetamol and ibuprofen tablets for her.

Examination

There is an obvious dinner-fork deformity to her right wrist with associated bruising and swelling. You cannot see any abrasions or puncture wounds. Assessment of the median, ulnar, radial nerves and wrist pulses is normal. Screening examination of the hand including scaphoid and elbow is normal.

| Investigations
| • AP and lateral radiographs of the right wrist are performed (Figures 48.1 and 48.2).

Questions

1. What is the diagnosis?
2. How are you going to manage this injury?
3. What methods of analgesia can you use to help with the reduction?

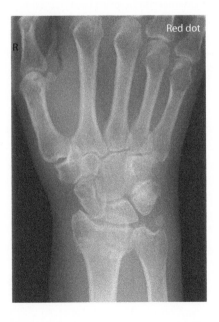
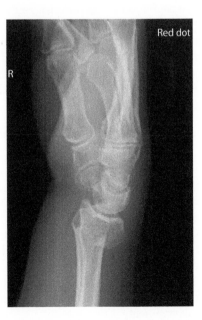

Figure 48.1 AP radiograph of the right wrist.

Figure 48.2 Lateral radiograph of the right wrist.

DISCUSSION

This lady has a closed distal radius and ulnar styloid fracture. This is a very common injury classically caused by falling onto an outstretched hand breaking a fall.

When taking the history, you should ascertain the dominant hand, premorbid function, occupational status and hobbies as these may influence management.

Fracture patterns can be variable and hence these injuries need careful evaluation both clinically and radiologically as this guides management. The Frykman classification system is used by orthopaedic specialists to grade injury (type I–VIII.)

This patient has a simple Colles type fracture, which may be treated with closed reduction in the ED and immobilisation in a plaster of paris backslab. Adequate analgesia is essential for proper reduction and good patient experience, and there several options:

1. Inhaled analgesia such as Entonox (nitrous oxide and oxygen) or Penthrox (methoxyflurane) may be adequate for minimally displaced fractures requiring the smallest of interventions to improve position.
2. Biers' block is used in certain departments. It is a regional block technique performed by placing an inflated double tourniquet on the arm and then injecting a measured dose of intravenous local anaesthetic (prilocaine) into the injured side.
3. Haematoma blockade is probably the most commonly used regional anaesthetic technique in the United Kingdom for distal radius fractures. Under strict aseptic conditions with skin prep and sterile drapes, local anaesthetic (lidocaine or bupivacaine) is injected directly into the fracture site. Correct placement is confirmed by first aspiration of 'haematoma'. Safe doses of local anaesthetic must be observed with typically 10–15 mL of 1% lidocaine being used depending on body weight. The block is allowed to develop for around 20 minutes, after which the reduction may be carried out. Equipment must be on hand in case of local anaesthetic toxicity, but with proper training and local protocol this is rare.
4. Procedural sedation may also be used but requires a trained operator and the appropriate monitored environment.

Reduction of the fracture is a straightforward process. You will need two assistants – one to help with the reduction and one to plaster.

1. Position the patient sitting up, with the shoulder abducted to 90 degrees and the elbow flexed to 90 degrees and the palm prone. Ask an assistant to gently hold the arm and provide counter traction. Take care when handling fragile skin in older patients.
2. Grasp the hand and slowly apply traction in the long axis of the radius. The key here is to slowly apply force over 5–10 minutes to overcome the patient's muscles and disimpact the fracture.
3. Slightly dorsiflex the distal fragment to unhinge the periosteum whilst maintaining traction and then bring the distal fragment downwards to restore normal anatomical alignment.
4. Maintain traction and ask your second assistant to apply a plaster of Paris backslab extending from the metacarpal heads to around 6 cm below the elbow joint. The wrist should be left either in a neutral position or slightly volar flexed. Gently compress the fracture site as the plaster hardens to provide additional support.
5. Document the neurovascular status post reduction and perform check radiographs.

The patient should be assessed by physiotherapists and occupational therapists prior to discharge, and should be given a sling for support and written instructions for plaster care and follow-up in the local fracture clinic.

These fractures do have a significant rate of movement, and the patient should be counselled regarding this. If the reduction is not adequate, the fracture may need re-manipulation either in the ED or in theatre and specialist help should be enlisted. Some fractures, particularly multi-fragmentary ones, are inherently unstable and may be better suited to operative methods of fixation.

 Key Points

- Take a comprehensive history including mechanism of injury, hand dominance, pre-morbid functional status, occupation and history.
- Always assess the joints above and below as there may be associated radial head fractures and carpal bone injury.
- Closed reduction should be performed in a strict protocolised manner in accordance to local guidelines.
- Seek specialist advice with complex fracture patterns, intra-articular fractures, inadequate reductions, open fractures and concomitant neurovascular injury.

History

A 22-year-old male software engineer presents to the Emergency Department. He was involved in a bar fight last night. He tells you that he punched a man in self-defense and then went home. When he woke up this morning, he noted that his right hand was swollen and painful on all movements. He does not complain of any other injury. The triage nurse has removed all rings from his hand.

Examination

On examination of his hand, significant swelling over the dorsal aspect of the metacarpals is noted. There are no defects or bite marks to the skin. He has a full range of flexion and extension of the fingers without scissoring or rotational deformity. Assessment of his median, radial and ulnar nerves and pulses is normal. Screening assessment of the wrist including scaphoid and elbow is normal.

 Investigations

- AP and lateral oblique radiographs of the hand are performed (Figure 49.1a and b).

Questions

1. How should you manage this injury?
2. What information will you give him regarding return to work and function?
3. How would your management differ if he had a 'fight-bite' injury?

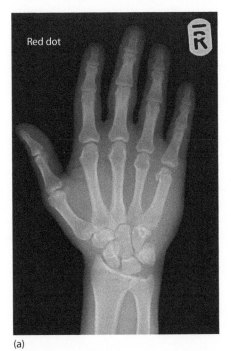

(a)

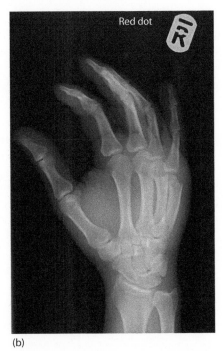

(b)

Figure 49.1 (a) AP and (b) lateral radiograph of the right hand.

DISCUSSION

This man has a fracture of the 5th metacarpal bone neck or a Boxer's fracture. It is a common injury often seen in young men and caused by high kinetic transfer through a closed fist.

Like all hand and wrist injuries, careful assessment is required. History should be thorough and include occupational status, hand dominance and hobbies, and should be extended to capture psychosocial aspects such as anger problems or possible domestic violence. The patient's recollection may be clouded by drugs or alcohol at the time of injury or circumstances surrounding the injury may not be intentionally disclosed. Clinical evaluation should cover examination of each finger in turn with assessment of bone, tendon and nerves at each joint. Look for rotational deformity or scissoring on finger flexion as this is an indication for operative fixation.

Should there be swelling at the base of the metacarpals, look for fracture dislocation at the carpometacarpal (CMC) joint on a true lateral radiograph. They are often subtle and so missed. This usually needs reduction and surgical fixation.

Fractures through the 5th metacarpal neck are inherently unstable as most are transverse. Volar angulation of up to 40 degrees at the neck is acceptable by most hand surgeons for conservative treatment. Attempts may be made to manipulate the fracture prior to immobilisation under regional block. There is no consensus on the best form of immobilisation, and options include simple neighbour strapping, ulnar gutter splints or a backslab with the wrist extended to 30 degrees and the fingers flexed to 90 degrees at the metacarpophalangeal joints (the Edinburgh position). Local orthopaedic guidelines should be followed.

A high arm sling is important post-immobilisation as there is a significant amount of associated soft tissue swelling and the patient referred to fracture clinic. Patients should be advised that they may have an alteration in their knuckle contour but function is good with hand physiotherapy. Indications for operation include rotational or scissoring deformity, fracture dislocations, open fractures, severe angulation and infected wounds.

If the patient sustains a bite injury at the same time, this is termed a 'fight-bite'. Clinically, this may vary from a small abrasion to a deep wound. Check the radiographs carefully for any tooth fragments embedded in the hand. Organisms from the mouth flora may include *Streptococcus viridans, Staphylococcus aureus, Eikenella* and *Fusobacterium*. The wound will need generous washout, debridement and broad-spectrum antibiotics (e.g. co-amoxiclav) along with tetanus immunoglobulin and/or vaccine as appropriate. Do not routinely close the wounds in the Emergency Department due to the high risk of infection. The patient will also need risk stratification, testing and immunisation against blood borne pathogens (hepatitis B, HIV) as per locally agreed protocols.

 Key Points

- Careful history taking and clinical assessment are vital in these patients.
- Most 5th metacarpal neck fractures can be managed conservatively.
- Follow-up and hand physiotherapy are essential for rehabilitation.
- Fight-bite injuries should be assessed for local infection and risk stratified for blood bourne infections.

CASE 50: CAT BITE

History

A 21-year-old man attends the Emergency Department after being bitten by his cat 3 days ago. He was feeding his cat when it bit him on the fingers. Since then his fingers have become progressively swollen and now there is pus leaking out of the wounds. The pain is unbearable and he cannot open his hand at all. He was born in the United Kingdom and was fully immunised as a child. The cat was purchased in the United Kingdom from a reputable breeder.

Examination

Vital signs: temperature of 38.9°C, blood pressure of 123/65, heart rate of 125 bpm, respiratory rate of 26, 99% O_2 saturations on air.

The patient looks unwell. The palm and fingers are diffusely swollen with clear puncture wounds to the index, middle finger and the thumb. On palpation, there is pain along the flexor tendons and passively extending the fingers causes significant pain. There is a serpiginous line extending from the hand along the forearm to the elbow.

 Investigations

- AP and lateral oblique radiographs of the hand do not demonstrate any fracture or foreign bodies, but significant soft tissue swelling is noted.

Questions

1. What is the likely diagnosis?
2. What is your initial management of this patient?
3. What would you do if this patient had not been immunised against tetanus?

DISCUSSION

This man has flexor tenosynovitis of the hand. Infection is usually caused by an inoculation event such as a cat bite due to their sharp needle like teeth. Classical presentation to the ED is around 24–72 hours post-injury.

Cat oral flora contains organisms such as *Staphyloccus aureus*, *Streptococcus viridans*, *Streptococcus pyogenes* and more importantly *Pasteurella multocida* and *Bartonella henslae*. These organisms cause a rapidly spreading infection through the finger soft tissues and the flexor tendon sheath resulting in accumulation of pus and compartment syndrome.

This patient has four defining clinical features known as Kanavel's signs:

1. Fusiform swelling of the finger
2. Fingers held in flexion
3. Significant pain on passive extension of the finger
4. Tenderness along the flexor tendon line

Once the diagnosis has been made, the patient should be resuscitated along standard sepsis guidelines with blood cultures, intravenous fluids and broad spectrum antibiotics such as co-amoxiclav or ceftriaxone. In case of penicillin allergy, consult local guidelines or seek advice from a microbiologist as macrolides may be ineffective. Take a wound swab in the ED for microscopy, culture and sensitivity.

The patient should be provided with adequate analgesia (opioids) and the affected limb elevated in a Bradford sling. He should be referred to the local hand surgeon for tendon sheath exploration and debridement in theatre.

Should infection be severe, pus may rupture into the mid-palmar space. Such infections are often associated with massive dorsal swelling of the hand and classically cause pain on passive finger extension. Again, this requires prompt surgical drainage.

Perform a thorough systemic examination as haematogenous spread can cause complications such as pneumonia, brain abscesses and infective endocarditis. You should also enquire about the tetanus immunisation status of the individual. If the patient has been immunised along the standard UK schedule with five vaccines, then the patient does not need a booster. If the patient's immunisation status is unknown or incomplete, the patient should receive human tetanus immunoglobulin as well as a tetanus vaccine at time of assessment. Patients will need their immunisation status clarified and vaccination completed as appropriate.

Consideration should also be given to other infectious agents such as rabies. This patient was injured by a UK-bred cat, but you may encounter patients presenting to the ED who have been abroad. Take a careful travel history including country of exposure, the animal (species, behaviour, vaccination status), number of days elapsed and any treatment abroad, and seek specialist advice. The Public Health England website has access to rabies maps and a risk stratification tool as well as contact information for virology advice.

Key Points

- Hand infections are an orthopaedic emergency and require thorough local and systemic clinical assessment.
- Take pus swabs prior to giving antibiotics in the ED.
- Ascertain tetanus immunisation status at time of injury and provide tetanus immunoglobulin and vaccine if there is partial or non-immunisation.
- Rabies risk stratification may be necessary if an animal bite wound was sustained abroad.

History

A 38-year-old motorcyclist is brought to the Emergency Department as a trauma call. He was travelling at 20 miles per hour and collided into the back of a stationary van. He was wearing full armoured riding gear and did not sustain a significant head injury. On scene, he removed his own helmet but could not stand. The attending paramedics transferred him onto a scoop stretcher and immobilised his cervical spine, applied a pelvic binder and brought him into the ED where you are waiting.

Examination

The patient is assessed along ATLS guidelines. Primary survey reveals an haemodynamically stable patient with significant pain to the left hip. Distal pulses are palpable in both legs.

Vital signs: blood pressure of 101/78, heart rate of 101 bpm, saturation of 100% on 15 L O_2, temperature of 35°C.

Investigations
• After an initial chest radiograph and point-of-care FAST scan, an AP pelvis radiograph is performed (Figure 51.1).

Questions

1. How do you classify pelvic fractures?
2. How are you going to manage the pelvic injury?
3. What other potential injuries do you need to assess for in the pelvic region?

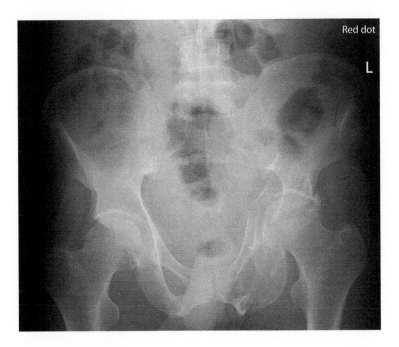

Figure 51.1 AP pelvis radiograph.

DISCUSSION

This patient has a fracture of the left iliac wing, acetabulum and pubic rami. Fractures of the pelvis are classified by the mechanism of injury. There are three main types:

1. AP compression (open book fractures)
2. Lateral compression injury
3. Vertical shear injury

Complex fracture patterns may also occur if the above mechanisms are combined.

Pelvic injuries may be associated with significant haemorrhage. There are two physical characteristics that account for this. Firstly, the internal pelvic volume roughly equates to an inverted cone. Increasing the radius of this cone, as in open book fractures, will greatly increase this volume. The other is the potential volume of the retroperitoneum. Even when intact it can accommodate the entire circulating blood volume. Bleeding in pelvic fractures is predominantly venous but may also be arterial. Clues may be elucidated on CT scan or by the site of injury.

Management of this patient should follow the step-wise approach as detailed by ATLS. Volume loss from bleeding should be replaced with either crystalloid or blood according to haemodynamic status. Permissive hypotension or balanced resuscitation may be employed to prevent dislodging primary clots. Whilst this is gaining more acceptance, local guidelines should be followed.

Often, a pelvic binder will have been applied by pre-hospital personnel, and this should not be removed until pelvic injury has been ruled out radiologically. Pelvic binders are most useful in 'open book' type injuries whereby they help to reduce pelvic volume.

Should the patient remain persistently hypotensive despite volume resuscitation and a binder, then the pelvis and retroperitoneum must be suspected as sources of ongoing blood loss once the other main sites have been excluded (chest, abdomen, long bones, open wounds).

Stable patients may be suited to angiographic embolisation in the interventional radiography suite. Unstable patients should be taken to a theatre by a trauma surgeon for pelvic packing and external fixation. Decision-making can be difficult as these patients are often young and may deteriorate suddenly (e.g. on the way to the interventional suite or CT scanner), and so senior support is advised from the outset.

The definitive management of pelvic fractures is surgical. They may be temporarily stabilised with an external fixator (either applied in theatre or the ED) to allow access to the abdomen and other life-threatening injuries to be treated before definitive operative management.

Open book fractures are also associated with bladder and urethral injuries. The presence of blood around the perineum, the urethral meatus or a high riding prostate should increase suspicion of this. Do not attempt to catheterise the patient. Obtain a urological opinion and perform a retrograde urethrogram to assess the urethra and the bladder first.

Key Points

- Pelvic fractures are associated with major trauma. Assess all patients according to ATLS guidelines.
- The mechanism of injury determines the fracture type and management.
- In the absence of other sources of haemorrhage, suspect pelvic or retroperitoneal blood loss in the persistently hypotensive patient.
- Assess the perineum carefully for potential bladder or urethral injury.

CASE 52: UNABLE TO STAND AFTER A FALL

History

A 90-year-old woman with dementia was found at her residential care home by the carer in the morning. It is unclear how long she has been on the floor. She cannot stand and has been brought in the Emergency Department complaining of pain in her right hip. She normally mobilises with a Zimmer frame and takes aspirin and a statin every night. There is no evidence of any head or neck injury.

Examination

Vital signs: temperature of 37.8°C, blood pressure of 130/60, heart rate of 121 bpm and irregular, respiratory rate of 24, 98% O₂ saturations on air.

Physical examination reveals a frail looking woman. There are no signs of head or neck injury and auscultation of the heart reveals a systolic murmur. Respiratory and abdominal examinations are unremarkable. Her right leg is shortened and externally rotated. There is a strong palpable dorsal pedis and posterior tibial pulse.

 Investigations
- Radiographs of the right hip are performed (Figures 52.1 and 52.2).

Questions

1. What is your initial management of the patient?
2. What forms of pain relief are suitable for this patient?
3. What are the operative management options for hip fractures?

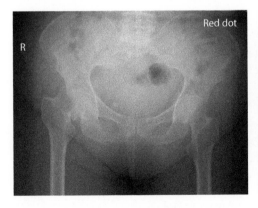

Figure 52.1 AP pelvis radiograph.

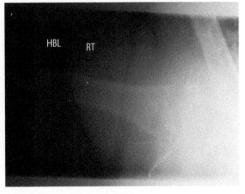

Figure 52.2 Lateral radiograph of the right hip.

DISCUSSION

This lady has a right neck of femur fracture. The initial management of this patient should follow standard trauma guidelines. Assessment should start with a top-down approach and you should assess for concurrent head and neck injury. A fall from standing can result in occult cervical spine fractures. If there is any doubt, then the patient should be immobilised and imaged to exclude injury. CT is the preferred imaging modality as plain radiographs may be hard to interpret in the context of degenerative disease.

This woman is noted to be in atrial fibrillation with a rapid ventricular rate and has a low-grade fever. Common sources of sepsis in older patients are the chest and urinary tract. Antibiotics should be provided after screening for infection and the appropriate samples taken. With regards to the atrial fibrillation, this may be driven by the sepsis or represent a new acute coronary syndrome. Serial 12-lead ECGs should be performed and troponin testing considered in this context. Rate control may be needed if the patient does not respond to fluid therapy and antibiotics. Rhabdomyolysis is another consideration as this patient was also found on the floor with a potential long lie overnight. Creatine kinase should be sent from the ED and the urine tested for myoglobinuria.

Titrated parenteral opioids (morphine) should be given early to these patients as this will help in transferring patients onto hospital beds, removing clothes and obtaining adequate radiographs. Once fracture has been confirmed, regional blockade in the form of a femoral nerve block or a fascia iliaca block may be instilled in the ED under ultrasound guidance and is now a widely accepted standard of care.

Most hospitals have a dedicated care pathway for elderly patients with hip fractures. It provides a standardised care bundle with specific goals including timely initial analgesia, radiographs, a checklist of blood investigations, urinary catheter insertion, skin checks, pressure-relieving mattresses, post-operative thromboprophylaxis and rehabilitation goals.

Assessment of these patients is multidisciplinary with co-assessment by an ortho-geriatrician being the norm. They provide expertise in rationalising medications, secondary bone protection therapy and guide rehabilitation, which may be prolonged in the context of frailty.

Operative fixation depends on the type of fracture. Hip fractures are divided into two main groups: intra- and extracapsular. Intracapsular fractures encompass any fracture to the femoral neck (subcapital, transcervical, basicervical), while extracapsular fractures lie at the level of the trochanteric line or below (intertrochanteric, subtrochanteric).

Within the joint capsule run the retinacular vessels, which are responsible for the majority of the blood supply to the femoral head. They are disrupted in intracapsular hip fractures, and the viability of the femoral head is threatened. Intracapsular fractures are usually treated with a hemiarthroplasty, especially in older patients. The damaged neck is excised in a theatre, and a titanium prosthesis is inserted into the proximal femur. The patient is immediately mobilised post-operatively to allow the metal work to embed.

Intertrochanteric fractures are the most common type of extracapsular fracture. The fracture is reduced in a theatre under fluoroscopic control on a traction table and fixed with a dynamic hip screw (DHS). This consists of a plate that is fixed to the proximal femur and a sliding screw that is passed along the neck of the femur into the femoral head. The patient is then mobilised post-operatively, which allows compression of the fracture and healing to occur.

Operative decision-making needs to consider the premorbid status of the patient and their ability to cope with the stress of anaesthesia as well as the individual fracture pattern. Should the operative risk be very high, the surgeon may elect to excise the fractured bone and let the hip joint form a pseudo-arthrosis. This is known as the Girdlestone–Taylor procedure.

Key Points

- Assessment of the elderly patient with a hip fracture should follow standard trauma guidelines.
- Look for and treat medical causes such as sepsis, delirium and acute coronary events as part of the pre-operative work up.
- Give early analgesia and consider local regional blockade as the gold standard of care.
- Operative fixation depends on the age of the patient and the type of fracture.

History

A 26-year-old man attends the Emergency Department. He has returned from a skiing trip where he injured his knee 2 days ago. He reports that he fell whilst skiing and cannot remember how he landed. At the time of injury, the knee was very swollen and he could not bear weight at all. He was seen at a sports clinic at the resort and had some x-rays performed. He was told that they did not show a fracture and was provided with crutches. Subsequently, the swelling has partially subsided but the knee does not feel stable on walking up and down stairs.

Examination

The left knee is swollen compared to the right. Range of movement is near normal (0–110 degrees) and he can do straight leg raise without a problem. Collateral ligament and meniscal tests are negative, but the anterior drawer test is positive. Gait is antalgic and the patient looks unsure of his steps. Distal neurovascular examination is normal.

Investigations
• AP and lateral radiographs of the left knee are performed (Figures 53.1 and 53.2).

Questions

1. What is the diagnosis and what does the radiograph show?
2. What injuries may be associated with this?
3. How are you going to manage this patient?

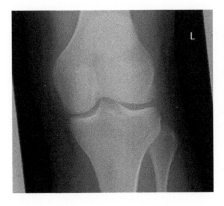

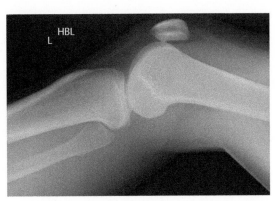

Figure 53.1 AP radiograph of the left knee.

Figure 53.2 Lateral radiograph of the left knee.

DISCUSSION

This man has a complete rupture of the anterior cruciate ligament (ACL). The history is typical of an ACL injury. This is often seen in younger patients and is associated with high-energy sports such as skiing, football or cycling.

Presentations may be delayed as patients may elect to self-care, or they are treated initially as 'soft tissue injuries' of the knee.

The radiographs in this case show a large lipohaemarthosis most evident in the lateral view extending into the suprapatellar pouch. The presence of this should raise suspicion of either an ACL tear or an occult fracture, and patients should be referred to the orthopaedic team. There may be an associated fracture of the lateral tibial plateau, and this is termed a 'Segond fracture'. Signs on plain radiograph may be subtle.

Definitive treatment depends on age, premorbid functional status and extent of injury (sprain, partial tear, complete tear). Minor sprains and incomplete tears of the ACL may be treated conservatively with physiotherapy and graded return to normal activity. Complete tears, as in this case, are usually treated operatively with ACL reconstruction with a patella tendon or hamstring graft. Exact timing of operation depends on the extent of injury, but it is usually performed on an urgent outpatient basis. The aim is to restore function and prevent any secondary injury to the articular surface or the menisci. This is followed by a period of rehabilitation and graded exercise. Prognosis and return to function are normally good in isolated injuries, but care should be taken not to reinjure the graft.

In cases where patients present early post-injury, examination may be limited due to pain. These individuals should receive follow-up in a fracture or sports injury clinic for re-evaluation once the pain of the initial injury has subsided usually in 7 days or sooner.

 Key Points

- Take a careful history in all knee injuries including the mechanism of injury and the timing of swelling.
- Examination should be systematic, and look for associated injuries.
- Plain radiographs may appear to be normal, but look carefully for the presence of effusions and fractures.
- Treatment of ACL injuries depends on the extent of the tear and the premorbid functional status of the patient.

History

A 75-year-old lady presents to the Urgent Treatment Center (UTC) with knee pain. She was out shopping earlier and fell over onto her knee. She heard a crack as she fell and was unable to stand. A shop assistant called the paramedics who applied a vacuum splint and have brought her into the UTC.

Examination

The right knee is swollen and deformed compared to the left. Range of movement is limited in all directions by severe pain, and the patient is most comfortable with the knee held in flexion. The dorsalis pedis and posterior tibial pulses are palpable, and there appears to be no distal neurological injury.

Investigations
• AP and lateral radiographs of the knee show a gross lipohaemarthosis and a tibial plateau fracture involving both medial and lateral sides with significant depression.

Questions

1. What is your initial management of this patient?
2. How are these injuries managed?
3. What are the potential complications of this injury?

DISCUSSION

This lady has a tibial plateau fracture. Assessment of the patient should follow standard trauma guidelines, and a rapid primary survey should be performed to rule out any occult injury. You should carefully examine the knee joint and the joint above (hip) and below (ankle). Should there be any concern that a second injury exists, perform radiographs to rule them out.

Tibial plateau fractures tend to have a bimodal distribution with age. In younger patients, they are often the result of high kinetic energy transfers (e.g. skiing, horse riding, falls from height and motor vehicles). Older patients tend to present with more insidious mechanisms. As bone density decreases with age, seemingly minor falls may produce severe fractures. The mainstay of injury is usually caused by the femoral condyles 'punching' down onto the tibial plateau.

When assessing these patients clinically, take care to assess and document the following:

1. *Knee stability* – In 10% of cases, there may be concomitant injury to the soft tissue structures of the knee (cruciate and collateral ligaments, menisci). Assessment may be difficult due to pain.
2. *Neurovascular status* – Severely displaced fragments may cause injury to the popliteal artery and the common peroneal nerve.
3. *Compartment status* – All injuries should be assessed for potential compartment syndrome, although this tends to be limited to those with high kinetic energy type injuries.

Subtle tibial plateau fractures are often missed in the ED and may be sent home inadvertently particularly in younger patients. Look carefully for the presence of a lipohaemarthrosis on the lateral view when assessing knee radiographs. This usually indicates occult injury and further investigation is warranted (CT or MRI).

Radiologically, tibial plateau fractures are graded using the Schatzsker classification (type I–VI) and are characterised by the degree of depression or displacement and the number of sides involved (lateral, medial, both). The most common form is type II (lateral plateau fracture with depression).

ED management should include adequate analgesia, immobilisation of the limb in an above-knee plaster of paris backslab, elevation and referral to the orthopaedic team. Most of these patients will need CT scanning to help delineate the injury and plan management as plain radiographs tend to underestimate the injury. Isolated fractures of the lateral side without significant depression (<4 mm) may be considered for conservative treatment especially in the older patient with comorbidities. Absolute indications for operative fixation are open fractures, neurovascular injury and compartment syndrome. A range of options are available for fixation, both internal (plate, screws, bone graft) and external (IIlizarov ring, hybrid devices), and specialist advice from a knee surgeon should be sought.

When assessing the older patient with minor trauma resulting in fracture, always investigate the possibility that this may be a pathological fracture (e.g. osteoporosis, malignancy). Multidisciplinary assessment with an ortho-geriatrician, occupational therapists and physiotherapists is invaluable. Care packages and social assessments may be needed for successful and safe discharge of these patients post definitive management.

Key Points

- Tibial plateau fractures may be subtle on plain radiographs and may be missed. Always look for the presence of a lipohaemarthosis.
- Remember to assess and document any associated soft tissue or neurovascular injuries.
- Refer these patients to the orthopaedic team for further imaging and definitive management.

History

A 19-year-old woman was out dancing last night. She was wearing high heels and fell over on the dance floor. She could walk immediately afterwards and went home. This morning, she has noted significant swelling to the lateral aspect of the ankle and has pain on weight bearing. She works in a retail shop and her manager has asked her to get it checked out.

Examination

There is a small swelling to the lateral aspect of the ankle just anterior to the lateral malleolus. Careful palpation reveals no bony tenderness to the distal 6 cm of both malleoli, the midfoot including the base of the 5th metatarsal, navicular, calcaneum and the forefoot. Ligamentous stress tests are normal as well as neurovascular examination. Screening examination of the knee is normal.

Questions

1. What is the diagnosis?
2. What are the indications for obtaining an x-ray?
3. What discharge advice are you going to give this woman?

DISCUSSION

This woman has a ligament sprain injury to her ankle. This type of presentation is typical to the Emergency Department and represents a sizable proportion of the workload in the urgent treatment or 'minors' areas.

Assessment of these patients is in two stages – assessment of the ankle and then assessment of the foot (hind-, mid- and forefoot) and knee. Take care to expose both legs to the knees and inspect carefully. There is often a small soft tissue swelling anterior to the lateral malleolus on the dorsum of the foot. This often correlates to a minor tear or sprain to the anterior talo-fibular ligament (ATFL) or the calcaneofibular ligament (CFL). This injury is classically referred to as a soft tissue injury to the ankle or a 'sprain'. The ankle is stable and the patient has minimal pain on weight bearing. Patients are often anxious with this type of injury and present to the ED seeking assessment.

Assessment should start at the ankle joint and the posterior bony part of the malleoli should be palpated down to the tip. Assess one side at a time. You should then extend your assessment through the calcaneum, midfoot and forefoot with particular attention to the navicular and the base of the 5th metatarsal. After bony palpation, you should test the lateral ankle ligaments and medial deltoid ligament to assess for widening and complete tears. Lastly perform a screening neurovascular examination and assess the knee, proximal fibula and gait.

Fractures to the base of the 5th metatarsal are often missed with ankle inversion injuries. The tendon of peroneus brevis runs on the lateral side of the ankle joint and inserts into the 5th metatarsal base. The tendon is very strong and inversion injuries can result in an avulsion fracture to the base.

Studies have shown that only around 15% of ankle x-rays demonstrate a fracture. This represents a significant proportion of patients who receive unnecessary radiation. The Ottawa ankle rules were developed to reduce the burden of radiographs by an estimated 30% and are validated primarily for use in adults. The 'rules' state that an ankle radiograph is indicated if any of the following conditions is met:

1. Pain to the posterior half or tip of the last 6 cm of the lateral malleolus
2. Pain to the posterior half or tip of the last 6 cm of the medial malleolus
3. Inability to walk independently at time of injury or assessment

The rules also state that a foot radiograph is indicated with patients with pain in the midfoot and any of the following:

1. Bony tenderness to the base of the 5th metatarsal
2. Bony tenderness to the navicular bone
3. Inability to walk independently at the time of injury or assessment

There can be inter-operator variability, but when properly applied, this clinical decision tool can demonstrate sensitivity of around 96%–99%.

Most sprains are suitable for conservative treatment, and the patient should be advised to rest the ankle, apply ice compresses and elevate in the first 48–72 hours. Some patients do benefit from compression (e.g. with double 'tubigrip' bandages or specialised supports), but evidence has not demonstrated a clear benefit. Crutches, with proper training on use, can be beneficial in moderating weight bearing in the acute stage.

Return to work and normal function are usually within a few days, but more severe sprains may take longer. The ability to weight-bear immediately post-injury is a good prognostic indicator of minor injury and prompt return to normal function. Self-directed ankle exercises should be encouraged and will prevent ankle stiffness and help reprogram damaged ankle proprioceptors. Recurrent sprains or more severe injuries should be referred for formal physiotherapy. In patients in whom complete ligamentous tears and ankle instability are suspected, orthopaedic referral and MRI imaging are advised.

Key Points

- Take a careful history and perform a systematic examination of the ankle and foot in patients with ankle injuries.
- The Ottawa clinical decision rule can help to decide which patients need imaging.
- Most patients will recover with rest, ice compresses and elevation.
- Patients with ankle instability or complete ligamentous tears should be referred to orthopaedic surgeons for further assessment.

History

A 30-year-old man was walking his dog in the park. The dog ran off chasing a rabbit and the man put his foot into a hole and fell over. He heard a snap as he fell and could not weight-bear at all. The paramedic crew removed his boot and applied a box splint and have brought him in as a priority call. They commented on a significant deformity to the ankle.

Examination

The ankle is visibly deformed and the patient is in significant pain. There is a triangle of stretched, pale white skin on the medial aspect of the ankle. The dorsalis pedis and posterior tibial pulses are palpable, and the patient tells you he can feel you touching his toes.

| Investigations
  • Immediate mobile radiographs are performed on the ankle (Figures 56.1a and b).

Questions

1. What is the diagnosis?
2. What is your immediate management of this patient?

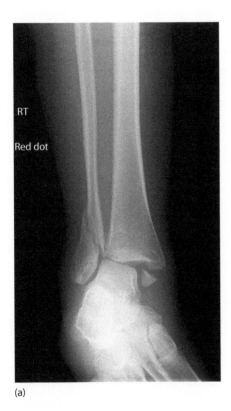

(a)

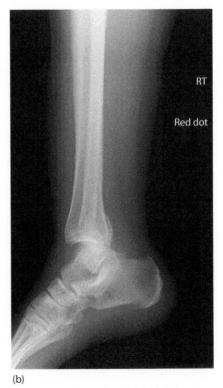

(b)

Figure 56.1 (a) AP and (b) lateral radiographs of the right ankle.

DISCUSSION

This man has a bimalloeolar fracture dislocation of the ankle with critical ischaemia of the skin. This is an orthopaedic emergency and requires prompt action. If the ankle is left in this position, the skin may tear converting a closed injury into an open one. The key here is to reduce the ankle with appropriate analgesia/sedation.

Rapidly assess the patient's foot and ankle in terms of direction of dislocation (almost always displaced laterally), neurovascular status and skin condition and move the patient into a monitored environment where you can give sedation. If the patient presents with an ischaemic foot, an open or contaminated wound, consult the orthopaedic team immediately. You will need at least three practitioners for the procedure – a sedationist, an 'operator' and a plaster technician or nurse. Most practitioners will elect to reduce the ankle without radiographs; however, should the opportunity exist to rapidly perform mobile radiographs, then this may guide your reduction. In any case, delay should be avoided.

Options for sedation may include inhaled agents such as Penthrox (methoxyflurane) or intravenous agents such as midazolam, ketamine or propofol which may be combined with analgesics such as fentanyl. The drugs used depends on the training and competence of the practitioner and patient choice. Analgesia and sedation should be given in a monitored environment by a trained practitioner after consenting the patient. The ankle is reduced by grasping the foot and pushing medially whilst dorsiflexing the foot into the anatomical position. Check pulses and skin condition post-reduction. Any abrasions or breaks in the skin should be carefully documented.

The foot and ankle should be held in the anatomical position and a below knee backslab applied. As the plaster hardens, take care not to let the ankle re-dislocate, and gentle pressure directed medially is helpful. Elevate the limb on soft stacked blankets. Isolated dislocations without fracture may require significant force to reduce the ankle, and adequate analgesia and sedation are essential.

Perform post-reduction radiographs and assess the extent of the injury – how many malleoli are involved (lateral, medial, posterior) and is there any talar shift? You should aim to reduce the ankle joint fully as malposition will encourage significant soft tissue swelling. You may need to re-manipulate the ankle until the talus is fully reduced within the mortise.

With isolated medial malleolus fractures or widening of the syndesmosis, perform radiographs of the whole lower leg to exclude a spiral fracture of the proximal fibula. This is termed a 'Maisonneuve' injury.

Ankle fracture dislocations need definitive operative management, and the patient should be referred to the orthopaedic team. The timing of surgery depends on the degree of soft tissue swelling. Early presentation with a swift reduction may be amenable to immediate open reduction and internal fixation. Those with significant swelling must wait until the surrounding tissues have recovered. Screen the patient for other injuries and remember to risk-stratify the patient for venous thromboembolism prophylaxis if prolonged inpatient immobilisation is anticipated.

	Key Points

- Carefully assess ankle fracture dislocations for neurovascular compromise and skin condition pre- and post-reduction.
- You may need to rapidly reduce the injury without radiographs if there is critical ischaemia of the skin.
- A trained practitioner should administer the sedation in a monitored and controlled environment.
- 'Open' injuries and those with non-viable ischaemic skin will need dual orthopaedic and plastic surgeon referrals.

GENERAL SURGERY AND UROLOGY

CASE 57: UPPER ABDOMINAL PAIN

History

A 43-year-old overweight male presents with an 8-hour history of worsening upper abdominal pain that radiates to his back. He has vomited twice. He denies any bowel or urinary symptoms. This is the first time the pain has lasted this long; usually it resolves within 2 hours. His comorbidities include diabetes milletus and hypertension. He smokes 30 cigarettes per day and 40 units of alcohol per week.

Examination

Vital signs: temperature of 38.7°C, heart rate of 108, blood pressure of 154/78, respiratory rate of 22, 96% saturation on room air. He has guarding in the right upper quadrant, but the abdomen is soft. Deep palpation on inspiration arrests his breathing. There is no organomegaly or distention.

Blood tests are pending.

Questions

1. What is the diagnosis?
2. What investigations does he require?
3. How would you manage him?

DISCUSSION

This patient has acute cholecystitis. He has a probable history of gallstones and is now febrile and Murphy's sign positive on examination.

Most patients with gallstones are asymptomatic. However, complications of gallstones range from biliary colic, whereby gallstones irritate or temporarily block the biliary tract, to acute cholecystitis, which is an infection of the gallbladder sometimes due to obstruction of the cystic duct. Gallstones can also become trapped in the common bile duct (choledocholithiasis) causing jaundice and potential ascending cholangitis, which refers to infection of the biliary tree. Ascending cholangitis classically presents with Charcot's triad of fever, right upper quadrant (RUQ) pain and jaundice. It can be life-threatening.

The majority of gallstones contain cholesterol but some contain pigment. Risk factors include pregnancy, elderly, obesity, haemolytic blood conditions (e.g. sickle cell disease, hereditary elliptocytosis) and certain ethnic groups (Hispanics, northern Europeans).

Biliary colic typically presents with wave-like RUQ or epigastric pain radiating to the back and is associated with nausea that starts after a heavy or fatty meal or at night. The patient moves around to get comfortable, as opposed to a peritonitic patient who lies still. The pain is usually self-resolving. The pain associated with acute cholecystitis is similar but lasts longer (>6 hours) and is usually associated with fever.

Murphy's sign is a sensitive examination sign for acute cholecystitis. Place your hand below the right costal margin in the RUQ and ask the patient to deeply inspire. If the gallbladder is inflamed, the patient will 'catch their breath' and experience pain.

Patients with epigastric or RUQ pain require a full blood count, renal and electrolyte screening, liver function tests (LFT), serum calcium and amylase/lipase level to rule out pancreatitis. In women of child-bearing age, a pregnancy test and urinalysis are vital. In biliary colic, the blood tests are usually normal, but in acute cholecystitis, there may be a leukocytosis and LFT derangement.

Jaundice does not occur in biliary colic and is not a common feature of acute cholecystitis. Its presence should raise suspicion for choledocholithiasis or Mirizzi syndrome whereby a gallstone in Hartmann's pouch or the cystic duct causes external compression of the bile duct.

The first-line investigation of choice for biliary colic or cholecystitis is ultrasonagraphy. This is quick and non-radiative (useful in children and pregnancy), and has a sensitivity of over 90%. It can also evaluate other causes of abdominal pain including the pancreas, liver, aorta and kidneys. The common features in cholecystitis are gallbladder wall thickening, distention and pericholecystic fluid. CT scanning of the abdomen is only indicated in diagnostic uncertainty. CT scanning does not identify gallstones that are isodense to bile, and so may provide false negative results.

Biliary colic requires supportive therapy in the form of adequate analgesia and anti-emetics, but does not require antibiotics. The patient should be counseled on dietary modification (avoiding fatty food and heavy meals). The patient should be referred to a general surgeon on an outpatient basis for consideration of a laparoscopic cholecystectomy.

Acute cholecytitis requires antibiotic therapy and admission under general surgery, who should decide whether to perform a 'hot' emergency cholecystectomy within 24–72 hours of admission. This shortens the hospital stay but can be associated with more surgical complications. Surgery may be indicated in cholecystitis complications including a perforated gallbladder causing peritonism or an empyema. Most patients will undergo an elective laparoscopic cholecystectomy once the inflammation has resolved.

Key Points

- Acute cholecystitis is associated with RUQ pain (>6 hours), fever and a positive Murphy's sign on examination.
- Ultrasonography of the abdomen and pelvis is the first-line investigation for gallstone disease.
- Management of acute cholecystitis includes antibiotics, fluids and dietary modification.

CASE 58: GRIPPING ABDOMINAL PAIN AND VOMITING

History

A 75-year-old lady presents with a 6-hour history of severe, gripping abdominal pain that peaks in waves. She has had eight episodes of bilious vomiting. She denies any urinary or bowel symptoms. Her co-morbidities include hypertension, osteoporosis and hypercholesterolaemia. She does not smoke or drink alcohol.

Examination

Vital signs: temperature of 36.7°C, heart rate of 108, blood pressure of 154/78, respiratory rate of 22, 97% saturation on room air.

Her abdomen is tender in the peri-umbilical region and distended. She has hyper-resonant bowel sounds but no organomegaly or peritonism. There is a mass extending into the inner thigh area that is irreducible and tender. The contents are tense and feel like bowel. The overlying skin is normal.

No blood or imaging investigations have been performed.

Questions
1. What is the diagnosis?
2. What investigations are appropriate?
3. How would you manage this patient?

DISCUSSION

This patient has small bowel obstruction (SBO), secondary to an incarcerated femoral hernia.

SBO is defined as a mechanical obstruction to the passage of contents in the bowel lumen. There can be complete or incomplete obstruction. The typical symptoms and signs of SBO are severe central cramping/griping (colicky) abdominal pain, nausea and vomiting and high-pitched bowel sounds. The interval between episodes of pain becomes longer as the site of obstruction becomes more distal. Constipation and distention are later signs. The signs of paralytic ileus include lack of bowel sounds (as opposed to hyperactive bowel sounds seen in true obstruction), distention, nausea and vomiting. The abdominal pain associated with paralytic ileus also differs; it is mild and non-cramping.

There are many causes of SBO. They can be extramural (e.g. by a mass, adhesions of hernia), mural (e.g. tumour, Crohn's disease, diverticulitis) or intra-luminal (e.g. foreign body, stricture, intussusception). The commonest cause of SBO worldwide is incarcerated herniae, whereas the commonest cause in the Western world is adhesion secondary to previous abdominal surgery.

Examination should include inspection for post-operative scars as well as all the hernia orifices. Typically, an incarcerated hernia cannot be reduced, has tense contents and has normal overlying skin. A strangulated hernia is irreducible, with tenderness and erythema of the overlying skin, due to a compromised blood supply. This is a surgical emergency associated with a high mortality. The patient is typically in septic shock, with fever, lactic acidosis, leukocytosis and tachycardia due to tissue necrosis. Look for signs of dehydration, which may present as an acute kidney injury, high haematocrit or concentrated urine.

As abdominal radiography has a sensitivity of around 50%, first-line imaging in the Emergency Department is more commonly becoming a contrast enhanced CT scan of the abdomen and pelvis. This will show loops of bowel dilated >2.5 cm, and then normal or collapsed bowel distal to a transition point. CT imaging helps to identify an underlying cause of obstruction, as well as rule out other causes of abdominal pain. Complications of SBO can also be identified, such as bowel perforation or ischaemia. This information also helps surgeons plan their operation pre-operatively. It should be noted that post-operative adhesive bands cannot be visualised on CT scanning, so suspicion for this as a cause is elicited from the clinical history and examination.

Management includes nasogastric aspiration with free drainage to reduce distention and the risk of aspiration. Dehydration and electrolyte imbalances should be corrected with appropriate intravenous fluids and regular fluid input/output monitoring. Analgesia and anti-emetics are also appropriate. If the cause of SBO is adhesion, a 'drip and suck' conservative approach can be trialed for 24 hours. Indications for surgery are worsening abdominal pain, sepsis or peritonism.

As this patient has an irreducible, tender femoral hernia, this must be repaired urgently and a general surgeon should be involved from the outset. Remember to give broad spectrum antibiotics in the ED should perforation be suspected and fluid-resuscitate the patient appropriately.

	Key Points
	• Small bowel obstruction is commonly due to post-operative adhesions or an irreducible (incarcerated) hernia.
	• It presents colic (cramping) abdominal pain, vomiting with distention and constipation developing later.
	• Contrast enhanced CT scanning is more sensitive than abdominal radiographs. It also rules out other causes of abdominal pain and helps to identify the cause and anatomical site of obstruction.
	• Management of all patients should consider intravenous rehydration and electrolyte correction, nasogastric aspiration, analgesia and anti-emetics. Surgery is indicated if a hernia is the cause, or in adhesions where the patient fails medical management or has SBO complications.

History
A 37-year-old male fell onto his side whilst under the influence of alcohol. He injured his ribs during the impact and has been acutely short of breath since the injury. He is a heavy smoker and drinks alcohol excessively. He denies any other medical or surgical history.

Examination
His respiratory rate is 28, peripheral oxygen saturation is 92% on room air, pulse is 103, blood pressure is 124/68 and temperature is 36.4°C. He has unilateral left-sided decreased chest expansion and breath sounds. There is marked bruising and tenderness across the left lower six ribs. The remainder of his examination is unremarkable.

 Investigations
* A mobile chest radiograph is performed in the resuscitation room (Figure 59.1).

Questions
1. What is the diagnosis?
2. What investigations are required?
3. How would you manage this patient?

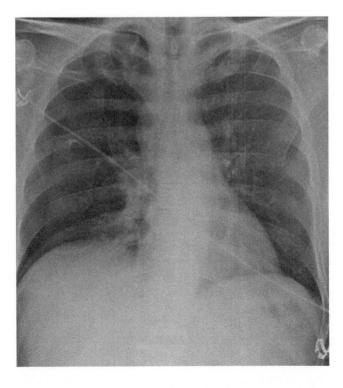

Figure 59.1 AP mobile chest radiograph performed in the resuscitation room.

DISCUSSION

This patient has a traumatic right-sided pneumothorax. A pneumothorax is a collection of air within the pleural space. There are four categories to be aware of: primary spontaneous pneumothorax (PSP), secondary spontaneous pneumothorax (SSP), traumatic pneumothorax and tension pneumothorax.

A traumatic pneumothorax, as seen in this patient, may be caused by a sharp spicule of bone injuring the pleura; if a blood vessel is injured, a haemothorax may develop concurrently. If a rib is broken in two places and the patient is in respiratory distress, inspect for a flail chest, whereby the segment of rib between the fracture lines is drawn inwards during inspiration and pushed outwards in expiration. A flail chest requires cardiothoracic surgical input to decide whether conservative or surgical management is appropriate.

Managing a traumatic pneumothorax should follow Advanced Trauma Life Support (ATLS) principles including performing a full primary and secondary survey to assess for other associated injuries such as splenic lacerations as in this case with left-sided trauma. The patient should have a two-wide bore cannulae inserted, a full set of blood tests including clotting and group and save, chest radiograph and a point-of-care ultrasound (eFAST) scan.

Most traumatic pneumothoraces are managed surgically with the insertion of a large (28–32F) caliber intercostal drain. This is placed in the fourth or fifth intercostal space, on the anterior–axillary line, and must be connected to an underwater seal. Antibiotic prophylaxis should be considered in all patients requiring a chest drain for a traumatic pneumothorax as per BTS guidelines. A chest radiograph should be performed afterwards to check drain placement.

If a patient continues to have respiratory compromise post-insertion, review drain placement (is it far enough?) and seal along with a full chest examination and review of the chest radiograph. It is possible for drains to fall out of position and the patient develop a tension pneumothorax.

A tension pneumothorax is a life-threatening emergency, which occurs when the intrapleural pressure exceeds the pressure in the lung. There is usually total collapse of the lung with compression of the mediastinum and inferior vena cava. This compromises venous return and cardiac output. Clinically this manifests as a diaphoretic patient who is agitated and gasping for breath. Clinical examination would show absent breath sounds on the affected side and tracheal deviation on the opposite side. A tension pneumothorax requires immediate decompression using a needle thoracostomy in the second intercostal space, mid-clavicular line using a 14G IV cannula. If there is a chest drain in situ, consider removing the retaining sutures and drain, and place a gloved finger into the thoracostomy space to re-open then tract. When the patient is settled, re-insert a chest drain and perform a radiograph to check the position. The patient may have developed a tension chest as the air leak may be bigger than the rate of drainage, and you may need to upsize the drain or insert multiple drains. Always call for senior help in these cases as early as you can.

Bear in mind that rib fractures can be very painful for several weeks. A local anaesthetic intercostal nerve block is an effective method of relieving acute pain. Thoracic epidurals may also be considered if offered by your local hospital. Regular chest physiotherapy and gentle mobilisation will help prevent secondary chest infection, but take care to ensure the drain does not move or fall out. This patient will also need counselling for his alcohol misuse and offered rehabilitation as well as nicotine, thiamine and chlordiazepoxide replacement to prevent delirium tremens whilst an inpatient.

 Key Points

- A pneumothorax is a collection of air within the pleural space.
- Assess all patients with traumatic pneumothoraces along ATLS guidelines.
- Look carefully for associated injuries.
- Most traumatic pneumothoraces or haemopneumothoraces are managed surgically with insertion of a wide bore intercostal drain.

History

A 62-year-old male presents to the Emergency Department (ED) with severe epigastric abdominal pain. The patient describes the pain as 'agonising' and 10/10 in severity. It started suddenly after a heavy evening meal, which was associated with a large amount of alcohol consumption.

His past medical history includes gastro-oesophageal reflux disease, for which he uses omeprazole 40 mg once a day for the last 10 years. He also regularly takes ibuprofen for osteoarthritis of the knee. He smokes 15 cigarettes per day and drinks 30 units of alcohol per week.

Examination

The patient is lying still on the bed with his legs pulled towards his chest, in the foetal position. His abdomen is distended, rigid to palpation with voluntary guarding in the epigastrium and absent bowel sounds. Percussion demonstrates a tympanic abdomen.

His pulse is 115, blood pressure is 103/62, respiratory rate is 28, SpO_2 is 94% on room air and temperature is 38.5°C.

Questions

1. What is the diagnosis?
2. What investigations would you request in the ED?
3. How would you manage this patient in the ED?

DISCUSSION

This patient has a perforated peptic ulcer. Differential diagnoses in this case would include acute pancreatitis (alcohol or gallstone due to age), perforated duodenal ulcer, perforated diverticulum/appendix, mesenteric ischaemia, inferior myocardial infarction and ruptured abdominal aortic aneurysm (AAA).

Immediate onset pain usually signifies a rupture or occlusion of an organ, whereas more insidious onset tends to be infective or inflammatory in origin. This should not be relied on as an absolute indicator, and a full history and examination should be performed.

In this case, the patient has acute onset severe upper abdominal pain, absent bowel sounds and signs of septic shock (tachycardia, hypotension). The patient also has board-like abdominal rigidity (involuntary muscle guarding) due to peritonitis. The patient usually lies completely still in the foetal position on the bed as movement is excruciatingly painful. Large doses of opiate analgesia are often needed at abating the pain, and this is a cardinal sign.

The history is not usually a reliable differentiator, but classically the difference in symptoms between gastric and duodenal ulcers is that gastric ulcers cause increased pain or indigestion on food ingestion, whereas duodenal ulcer reduces pain. Risk factors include gastro-oesophageal reflux disease, *H. pylori* infection, smoking or alcohol excess, prolonged steroid or non-steroidal anti-inflammatory drug (NSAID) use.

A perforated peptic ulcer tends to raise both the white cell count and serum amylase, the latter due to absorption from the peritoneum into the blood stream. A quick test in the ED includes an erect chest radiograph, which may show free air under the diaphragm, although around a quarter of patients with perforation do not radiographically demonstrate a pneumoperitoneum. Contrast enhanced CT scanning of the abdomen is a more sensitive investigation and can be performed relatively quickly nowadays. It helps confirm the diagnosis of a perforation as well as its underlying cause. It also guides surgical management by delineating the level of the perforation; upper GI perforations are generally associated with more gas than fluid, whereas lower GI perforations have more fluid than gas.

Management should include early goal directed therapy of sepsis, keeping the patient nil by mouth, nasogastric tube insertion and aspiration of gastric contents, urinary catheter insertion with hourly urinary output monitoring and opioid analgesia. Crucially, they also require early administration of broad-spectrum antibiotics as per local hospital guidelines. A third-generation cephalosporin and metronidazole will provide good cover against aerobic and anaerobic bacteria. Pre-operative antibiotics also reduce the chance of post-operative wound infection.

The surgical team should be involved from an early stage as should the critical care team if warranted by the patient's condition. Should the patient not respond to volume resuscitation, then an arterial line should be placed and vasopressors started in the ED. The patient will need to be adequately resuscitated and optimised prior to anaesthesia and surgery.

 Key Points

- A perforated peptic ulcer is a surgical emergency that presents with upper abdominal pain, decreased or absent bowel sounds and signs of septic shock.
- Management should follow early goal directed therapy of sepsis including early administration of broad spectrum antibiotics and fluid resuscitation.
- Prompt surgical intervention is key.

History

A 57-year-old male presents with a 12-hour history of worsening, constant left iliac fossa pain associated with fever. He suffers from constipation, which has become worse over the past week, but denies any urinary symptoms or weight loss. His past medical history includes asthma and hypercholesterolaemia.

Examination

He is saturating at 96% on room air, and his respiratory rate is 26, heart rate is 104, blood pressure is 115/65 and temperature is 38.3°C. Abdominal examination demonstrates left iliac fossa tenderness and guarding. Rectal examination is painful but no masses are appreciated.

Questions

1. What is the diagnosis?
2. What investigations are required?
3. How would you manage this patient?

DISCUSSION

Diverticular disease (diverticulosis) is a condition where small outpouchings (diverticula) develop in the large bowel, most commonly the sigmoid colon. Diverticulitis is an infection of the diverticulae, which may be caused by obstruction by faecoliths. This may progress into a pericolic abscess (outside the bowel), which can cause peritonitis if it ruptures. The infection is caused by a mixture of aerobic bacteria (*E. coli, Enterobacter, Klebsiella* and *Proteus*) and anaerobic (*Bacteroides* and *Clostridium*) gut flora.

The outpouching (diverticululm) is a herniation of mucosa and submucosa. It occurs where there is weakness in the bowel wall at the points where nutrient blood vessels enter. Its incidence increases with age, affecting 50% over 60 years old. However, only up to 20% of these people become symptomatic. It is more common in people with low fibre diet and chronic constipation.

Patients with sigmoid diverticulitis present with constant aching left lower quadrant abdominal pain, change in bowel habit (mostly constipation but sometimes diarrhoea) and fever. Patients may have nausea and anorexia.

Classically, abdominal examination demonstrates left iliac fossa tenderness and guarding, hence giving rise to the term 'left-sided appendicitis'. Rectal examination is painful but can help exclude a rectal or low colon cancer.

Blood tests will show a leukocytosis and raised inflammatory markers, but these can be normal in a small proportion of patients. Renal function testing is important to look for an acute kidney injury or electrolyte disturbance in those with altered bowel function. Urinalysis may show a microscopic haematuria, and this can represent irritation of the underlying ureter. A pregnancy test is compulsory in women of childbearing age. You should take blood cultures before administering antibiotics as this may help guide ongoing therapy.

In the acute setting, contrast enhanced computed tomography (CT) of the abdomen and pelvis is the best method for diagnosing diverticulitis and its complications including abscess, perforation or obstruction. Plain supine abdominal films can diagnose bowel obstruction or ileus, but are generally poor at diagnosing diverticulitis. If there is clinical concern about bowel perforation, an erect chest radiograph should be performed to look for pneumoperitoneum.

Mild uncomplicated acute diverticulitis can be managed as an outpatient with oral antibiotics that cover gut flora (e.g. co-amoxiclav or ciprofloxacin and metronidazole). Clinical improvement is usually seen in 2–3 days of treatment, and patients should be advised to adhere to a clear liquid diet during this time. If symptoms do not resolve or worsen, then advise patient to return to the Emergency Department. Unwell patients, the elderly or those with very high inflammatory markers should be admitted for inpatient intravenous antibiotic therapy.

Those with diverticular perforation should be resuscitated in the ED along standard sepsis protocols (antibiotics, fluids, inotropes, catheter, NG tube) and will need surgical intervention in the form of an exploratory laparotomy, washout and a de-functioning colostomy. The colostomy is reversed later after the patient has recovered from the acute episode, usually 3 to 6 months later. Perforation carries a high mortality rate, and early involvement of critical care specialists is key.

Key Points

- Diverticulitis describes an infection of outpouchings in the large bowel and may present with left iliac fossa pain, fever and change in bowel habit.
- Management should follow early goal directed therapy in treating sepsis with broad spectrum antibiotics covering intestinal flora.
- Consider early CT scanning if complications such as abscess, perforation or obstruction are suspected.
- Surgical teams should be involved early in the care of the unwell patient.

CASE 62: ACUTE SEVERE LEG PAIN

History

An 84-year-old male with a background of atrial fibrillation, type 2 diabetes mellitus and hypertension presents with acute right leg pain that started 3 hours ago. He has never experienced such pain before and is frightened that he cannot feel his leg. He is a lifelong smoker and drinks 40 units of alcohol per week. He has never had an operation before and takes aspirin, metformin and anti-hypertensives.

Examination

The gentleman has central obesity with a BMI of over 35. The right leg is pale, is cold and lacks sensation or pulses below the level of the knee. He is unable to actively flex or extend his knee or ankle. Passive ankle dorsiflexion is excruciatingly painful. Examination of the left leg is unremarkable – his radial pulse is irregular, but he has normal heart sounds. His abdominal examination is also normal. His temperature is 36.2°C, pulse is 108, blood pressure is 168/87, respiratory rate is 26 and oxygen saturation is 90% on room air.

Questions

1. What is the diagnosis?
2. How would you manage this patient?
3. What are your concerns?

DISCUSSION

Acute ischaemia describes the occlusion of an artery. It is most commonly the result of a thrombo-embolus in a patient with atrial fibrillation, but it may also be caused by in situ thrombosis of an atheromatous lesion. Vascular trauma and aneurysms are other causes.

The characteristic six Ps of acute arterial occlusion are pain, pulseless, paralysis, paraesthesia, pallor and 'perishingly cold'. The pain is of acute onset, and the patient can usually tell you where and when it started. Muscle tenderness may be a sign of ischaemia or compartment syndrome.

Clinical assessment should look for a cause. For example, an irregularly irregular pulse and electrocardiogram can confirm atrial fibrillation, a pulsatile expansile abdominal mass indicates an aortic aneurysm and presence of pulses in the contralateral limb may suggest a thromboembolism. A hand held doppler is a useful quick bedside examination technique and may demonstrate reduced or absent pulses or a reduced Ankle Brachial Pressure Index (ABPI). The imaging modality of choice is duplex ultrasonography or (CT) angiography and helps to establish the site of vascular occlusion as well as distal vessel patency and collateral formation.

After making the diagnosis in the emergency department, insert two cannulae into the patient. Blood should be drawn for full blood count (polycythaemia, platelets), urea and electrolytes (acute kidney injury), creatine kinase (rhabdomyolysis), clotting (coagulopathy, baseline) and group and screen as well as a venous blood gas (lactate, blood sugar). Administer intravenous opioids titrated to pain and fluid-resuscitate the patient. Start an intravenous heparin infusion and contact the local vascular service. Potential management options include angioplasty of the lesion, thrombectomy, catheter directed thrombolysis and bypass grafting. Age, premorbid status, the location and length of the lesion play important roles in determining the best option for the patient, and management is best guided by an experienced vascular surgeon. Should the limb be unsalvageable (long ischaemia time, severe co-morbidities, severe infection), then you may need to proceed to amputation. Very co-morbid and elderly patients who may not survive operation or interventional radiology and who have a poor prognosis may be palliated.

After treatment of the acute lesion, patients must optimise control of blood pressure, diabetes mellitus, hypercholesterolaemia as well as lifestyle modifications such as smoking cessation, limiting alcohol consumption, weight loss and increasing exercise.

 Key Points

- The characteristic six Ps of acute arterial occlusion are pain, pulseless, paralysis, paraesthesia, pallor and perishingly cold.
- Acute ischaemia is most commonly the result of a thromboembolus in a patient with atrial fibrillation.
- Start intravenous heparin in the Emergency Department and speak to a vascular surgeon immediately.
- Definitive management options include angioplasty, thrombectomy, catheter directed thrombolysis, bypass operation and amputation.

CASE 63: ABDOMINAL PAIN AND NAUSEA

History

A 19-year-old male presents with lower right-sided abdominal pain that is constant. It started 24 hours ago with cramping abdominal pain. He is off his food, feeling sick and feverish. He has had several episodes of loose stools over the last 12 hours.

He does not have any other medical problems and has never experienced pain like this before.

Examination

His abdomen is soft, with tenderness in the right iliac fossa. There is no renal angle pain, abdominal mass or organomegaly. Scrotal and testicular examination is normal.

His temperature is 37.9°C, pulse is 105, blood pressure is 93/54, respiratory rate is 28 and oxygen saturation is 98% on room air.

 | Investigations
- Blood tests demonstrate WCC 18.1 and CRP 49. His urinalysis contains a trace of blood.

Questions
1. What is the diagnosis?
2. What investigations are appropriate? When would you perform a CT scan?
3. How would you manage this patient?

DISCUSSION

This patient has acute appendicitis. Obstruction of the appendix lumen results in a closed loop and inflammation; this can cause appendix necrosis and perforation. The commonest causes are lymphoid hyperplasia or a faecolith (appendicolith). Rarely it can be a presentation of a tumour such as appendiceal carcinoid tumour. The lifetime risk of developing appendicitis is 5%–10%, and it is the commonest cause of emergency abdominal surgery in the Western world.

Classically appendicitis is described as presenting with the following chronologically, but naturally there are deviations to this description:

- Periumbilical abdominal pain that is intermittent and cramping. This is due to referred pain.
- Nausea or vomiting – in appendicitis, pain classically precedes vomiting, whereas the opposite occurs in gastroenteritis.
- Anorexia.
- Low-grade fever.
- Migratory right iliac fossa (RIF) pain that is constant and intense (usually 24–48 hours after the onset of periumbilical pain). Pain localised to the RIF is due to local peritoneal irritation.

The most reliable sign on examination is tenderness over McBurney's point, defined as a point one-third of the distance from the umbilicus to the anterior superior iliac spine. Peritoneal irritation manifests as guarding and rebound tenderness.

The following special tests have a relatively low sensitivity. A positive Rovsing's sign refers to pressure over the left iliac fossa to causing peritoneal irritation and pain in the right iliac fossa. A retrocaecal appendix (seen in 60%–70% of patients) may produce a psoas sign (pain on flexing the hip against resistance, which irritates the retroperitoneal iliopsoas muscle). If the appendix lies in the pelvis (around 20%), the obturator sign may be positive (pain upon internal rotation of the leg with the hip and knee in flexion).

There are many causes of RIF pain, and the history and examination can provide clues as what the likely cause may be. The differential includes mesenteric adenitis, Meckel's diverticulum, perforated ulcer, urinary tract infection or pyelonephritis, renal colic, pancreatitis, inflammatory bowel disease flare, gastroenteritis and neoplasm. In women, consider additional gynaecological pathologies such as an ovarian torsion, tubo-ovarian abscess, pregnancy (or ectopic) and pelvic inflammatory disease.

Investigations should include blood tests for full blood count, renal function, electrolytes and C-reactive protein. Typically, there will be a leukocytosis and raised CRP if there has been enough time for it to rise. Blood cultures are appropriate if the patient is febrile or has signs of sepsis. A raised serum lactate, which is measured as part of a venous blood gas analysis, may demonstrate inadequate tissue perfusion as part of a septic picture.

Urinalysis will help rule out renal pathology such as urinary tract infection, pyelonephritis or renal colic. However, haematuria and pyuria can be seen in appendicitis causing ureteric inflammation. A urinary pregnancy test or serum beta-HCG test is essential in all women to exclude pregnancy. Appendicitis is the commonest general surgical emergency in pregnant women and may have an atypical presentation with pain anywhere in the right side of the abdomen (usually the right upper quadrant).

Ultrasonography can also be a quick form of imaging without radiation that helps to evaluate gynaecological pathology, although the appendix is not always visualised. Its sensitivity, specificity and accuracy are around 80%–90%, but this is user dependent. As it does not use radiation, it is useful in children and women who may be pregnant.

Contrast-enhanced computed tomography (CT) of the abdomen and pelvis is indicated if there is diagnostic uncertainty. This should be discussed with the radiologist, especially in young patients. Its sensitivity, specificity and accuracy are over 90%. In appendicitis, a CT scan will show periappendiceal fat stranding and fluid, a widened appendix diameter >6 mm and possibly an appendicolith. Abdominal radiographs do not have a high diagnostic yield and should not be performed as routine. A chest radiograph can exclude lung pathology and viscus perforation if this is suspected.

The mainstay of treatment of confirmed appendicitis is an appendicectomy, which may be open or laparoscopic. Appendiceal abscesses may be treated with prolonged antibiotics and then an interval appendicectomy. In a septic or peritonitic patient, early goal directed therapy should be instituted. This includes administering oxygen therapy if appropriate, broad-spectrum intravenous antibiotics within 3 hours of arriving in the Emergency Department and intravenous crystalloid fluid resuscitation for hypotensive or dehydrated patients.

Symptom management should include titrated intravenous opioids, intravenous anti-emetics and fluid. From an early stage, involve a General Surgeon as the mainstay of treatment is operative. Doing this early prevents appendiceal perforation and its complications. It is estimated that 25% of appendicitis will perforate 24 hours from the onset of symptoms, and 75% by 48 hours.

If the diagnosis is in doubt, further imaging or repeat examination of the abdomen as well as serial monitoring of the temperature and pulse are appropriate. It may become necessary to perform a diagnostic laparoscopy +/– appendicectomy if there is still diagnostic uncertainty. This is useful in women of childbearing age.

The commonest reason to visit the Emergency Department after an appendicectomy is wound infection, and for this reason, patients may be given a 7-day course of antibiotics post-operatively, especially if there was appendiceal perforation.

Patients with non-specific abdominal pain may be discharged if their history and examination are not suggestive of appendicitis, they do not have raised inflammatory markers and they have a normal urinalysis and negative pregnancy test. They should be warned to return if they develop worsening abdominal pain, nausea, anorexia, fever or migratory RIF pain.

If in doubt, obtain a senior opinion or treat the patient clinically with admission for observation and periodic re-examination.

The use of ambulatory surgical care is becoming more common, which allows well patients to return the next day and have repeat blood tests to see if inflammatory markers have risen and further imaging as indicated.

 Key Points

- An acute appendicitis presents with periumbilical abdominal pain that migrates to the RIF. This is associated with nausea or vomiting, anorexia, low-grade fever and tenderness over McBurney's point.
- Pregnancy and urinary tract infections should be ruled out especially in women.
- Confirmed appendicitis requires an appendicectomy.

History

A 55-year-old woman presents to the Emergency Department with a 2-day history of worsening right upper quadrant and epigastric pain that sometimes moves around to her back. The pain is now constant and is not relieved by paracetamol or ibuprofen. She has been feeling nauseous and has vomited on a few occasions. She has a history of diet-controlled type 2 diabetes and hypertension. She does not smoke and denies significant alcohol intake.

Examination

Vital signs: temperature of 37.2°C, blood pressure of 100/60, heart rate of 110 and regular, respiratory rate of 24, 95% O_2 saturation on air.

General examination reveals an ill-appearing woman who is in severe pain. Cardiorespiratory examination is normal, but the abdomen is very tender over the right upper quadrant and epigastrium. There is no guarding, rebound tenderness or organomegaly.

Questions

1. What is the differential diagnosis, and which do you think is the most likely diagnosis?
2. What investigations should be performed in the Emergency Department to confirm the diagnosis?
3. How would you manage the patient acutely?

DISCUSSION

The differential diagnosis of right upper quadrant and epigastric pain includes conditions affecting the upper GI tract, namely the oesophagus, stomach, duodenum and pancreas. Gastritis, peptic ulcer disease, biliary disease (e.g. gallstones, cholecystitis, cholangitis), pancreatitis and mesenteric ischaemia are the key conditions to consider in such cases, though it is also worth remembering that right basal pneumonia and inferior myocardial infarction can also mimic such symptoms. In this case, the history of right upper quadrant and epigastric pain radiating to the back points towards acute pancreatitis secondary to gallstones, and this is also supported by the presence of nausea and vomiting (seen in >90% of patients).

When suspecting a case of acute pancreatitis, there are three important questions to be answered, which will guide further investigation:

 i. How do you confirm the diagnosis?
 ii. What is the likely cause?
 iii. How severe is the disease?

Confirmation of the diagnosis requires at least two of the following: characteristic acute epigastric pain radiating to the back, elevated pancreatic enzymes and typical findings on imaging (usually CT). Common causes of pancreatitis are mechanical obstruction (gallstone disease, ampullary obstruction), toxins (alcohol, scorpion venom), drugs (steroids, thiazides), infection (mumps, coxsackie, CMV), metabolic (hyperlipidaemia, hypercalcaemia) and post-ERCP. Therefore, initial investigations that should be performed include renal function and electrolytes, full blood count, liver enzymes and amylase or lipase (the latter has a higher sensitivity, but may not be available in all departments). An abdominal ultrasound should also be arranged to look for gallstones. Point-of-care ultrasound performed by trained practitioners in the ED is useful in ruling out other causes abdominal pain that radiates to the back such as an abdominal aortic aneurysm. CT scanning may be considered if there is diagnostic uncertainty or if complications such as pancreatic necrosis or large pseudocyst are suspected.

Pancreatitis can be classified as mild, moderate or severe, based on the presence or absence of organ dysfunction (e.g. renal or respiratory failure) and/or local and systemic complications (e.g. pseudocyst, necrosis). There are also various scoring systems available that can predict disease severity and help select which patients require higher-level care and monitoring (e.g. in an intensive care unit). One model is the Ranson score, which is based upon five admission parameters (age, white cell count, blood glucose, LDH and AST) and additional six parameters after 48 hours (haematocrit, urea, calcium, pO_2, base deficit and fluid sequestration), with higher scores correlating with greater mortality.

There are three main facets that form the basis of the initial management of acute pancreatitis: (i) fluid repletion, (ii) pain control and (iii) nutrition. Aggressive intravenous hydration is required in all patients (taking into account any relevant cardiac history), with several litres typically needed in the first 1–2 days; the rate of fluid administration can be adjusted according to clinical and laboratory parameters (heart rate, blood pressure, urine output, renal function tests). Controlling pain with the use of strong opiates if required is important as it is the principal symptom for patients, and uncontrolled pain can worsen the systemic inflammatory response. Finally, most patients with pancreatitis require bowel rest, at least initially, in order to prevent aggravating inflammation via stimulation of pancreatic enzymes; nutrition can be resumed as pain allows and as the clinical state improves, but nutritional support (e.g. with nasojejunal feeding) is often required in severe cases and those where complications are present.

Key Points

- Epigastric pain is generally caused by conditions affecting the oesophagus, stomach or pancreas.
- Diagnosing pancreatitis requires at least two of the following: characteristic epigastric pain radiating to the back, elevated pancreatic enzymes and specific imaging findings on CT.
- Intravenous hydration, pain control and bowel rest are key in the early management of pancreatitis.

History

A 68-year-old man presents with a 1-hour history of severe left-sided loin to groin pain. He has never experienced such pain and denies any urinary or bowel symptoms. His comorbidities include hypertension, diabetes mellitus and chronic obstructive airway disease. He is a lifelong smoker of 20 cigarettes per day and drinks 30–40 units of alcohol per week.

Examination

His temperature is 35.9°C, pulse is 115, blood pressure is 89/48, respiratory rate is 24 and oxygen saturation is 94% on room air. Abdominal examination reveals a distended abdomen, which is diffusely tender and a pulsatile mass in the upper half.

Questions

1. What is the diagnosis?
2. What investigations are appropriate?
3. What is permissive hypotension?
4. How would you manage this patient?

DISCUSSION

This patient has an abdominal aortic aneurysm (AAA), which is defined as a dilatation of an artery to more than 50% of its normal diameter. This classically presents with a triad of abdominal pain, pulsatile abdominal mass and hypotension. However, it should be ruled out in all over-65-year-old patients with abdominal pain. Do not be lured into a diagnosis of renal colic in an older patient, without definitive imaging to rule out an AAA rupture.

The normal diameter of the infrarenal aorta is 2 cm, and therefore, an aneurysm will measure >3 cm. The commonest aetiology is atherosclerosis, which causes degeneration of the tunica media layer of the vessel. It is much more common in males than females. The biggest risk factor is smoking; other factors include hypertension, chronic obstructive pulmonary disease, family history and older age (>60). The risk of rupture increases with enlarging diameter due to Laplace's law, which describes an increase in vessel wall tension with an increase in diameter (wall tension = pressure × diameter).

The examination findings are classically a pulsatile, expansile mass. Ensure to palpate above the umbilicus but below the xiphisternum as the aorta bifurcates at the level of the umbilicus. Point-of-care ultrasound is now used routinely in most Emergency Departments to confirm the presence or absence of an aortic aneurysm. It is, however, limited in that it cannot reliably rule out a leak. It is also limited in the setting of obesity or overlying bowel gas, which may make significant portions of the aorta invisible. The gold standard imaging modality is a contrast enhanced CT scan of the aorta, which has a sensitivity of almost 100% and can help rule out other causes of abdominal pain if the diagnosis is uncertain. CT scanning can demonstrate impending rupture, contained leakage or frank rupture of the AAA.

Investigations should not delay emergency treatment. Place the patient in the resuscitation room, and place at least 2 14G cannulae. Take blood for full bood count, renal function and clotting, and cross-match at least 6 units of blood.

Consider activating the major transfusion protocol if the systolic BP is <90 mmHg or heart rate >110 bpm. This will speed up the laboratory's release of packed red cell, fresh frozen plasma, cryoprecipitate and platelets. Prepare to place a urinary catheter, arterial lines and central venous catheters should there be time.

Fluid-resuscitate the patient and consider using packed red cells as a first-line agent. Be careful not to raise the blood pressure too far as this may exacerbate a leak. The concept of permissive hypotension avoids aggressive fluid resuscitation, as a higher blood pressure will result in more bleeding. The aim should be for the lowest systolic blood pressure while maintaining vital organ perfusion. This is usually around 90 mmHg systolic. Pain control with intravenous morphine will also reduce wall tension and cardiac contraction.

A ruptured AAA has a 100% mortality unless immediately repaired. It requires immediate referral to a vascular surgeon and repair, either by open surgery or endovascular aneurysm repair (EVAR). EVAR involves femoral artery catheterisation and stent insertion.

Incidental or asymptomatic AAAs discovered in the Emergency Department also warrant referral to a vascular surgeon. Indications for repair include a male with an AAA >5.5 cm or female with an AAA >5 cm or rapid growth of more than 1 cm/year. Asymptomatic AAAs measuring 2–5.5 cm requires regular ultrasonography and vascular surgery outpatient input.

Key Points

- A ruptured AAA is a surgical emergency with 100% mortality if not immediately repaired. It classically presents with abdominal pain, pulsatile abdominal mass and hypotension.
- It should be ruled out in all patients over 65 years of age presenting with abdominal, loin or groin pain, especially if they have risk factors including smoking, hypertension, COPD or peripheral vascular disease.
- Point-of-care ultrasonography is a rapid and non-invasive investigation that can be used in unstable and stable patients.
- Treatment involves expedient management to a vascular surgeon who will decide on open surgery or EVAR.

CASE 66: RIGHT FLANK PAIN MOVING TO THE GROIN

History

A 30-year-old man presents to the Emergency Department with a 6-hour history of excruciating right-sided abdominal pain. The pain is over his right flank and comes in waves, with each episode lasting 30–40 minutes; it also occasionally moves towards his groin. He denies dysuria or visible haematuria. He has a history of Crohn's disease and has undergone extensive small bowel resection.

Examination

Vital signs: temperature of 36.7°C, blood pressure of 155/80, heart rate of 80 and regular, respiratory rate of 20, 96% O_2 saturation on air.

General examination reveals a slim man who is writhing in pain. He appears dehydrated, but cardiorespiratory examination is normal. The abdomen is tender on palpation of the right flank, with percussion tenderness over the right costophrenic angle.

 Investigations

- Urine dipstick is positive for blood (2+), but negative for nitrites and leukocytes.

Questions

1. What is the likely diagnosis, and what risk factors does this patient have for this?
2. What investigations should be performed in the ED?
3. How would you manage the patient? Does the patient need admission, and is there a need to seek input specialist?

DISCUSSION

Severe unilateral flank pain that comes and goes in waves and that radiates towards the groin is typical of ureteric colic, where the symptoms correlate with the passing of a kidney stone from the renal pelvis into the ureter. Pain is very common, with other features including haematuria, nausea, vomiting, urinary symptoms (frequency, dysuria) and testicular or penile pain. Pain is thought to result when the stone becomes lodged in the ureter, with flank pain thought to result from upper urinary tract obstruction and groin or pelvic pain arising from obstruction at the lower ureters or vesicoureteric junction (VUJ).

Risk factors for nephrolithiasis include personal and family history of stone disease (up to 30% of patients with kidney stones have a recurrence within 5 years), urinary tract infections, inadequate hydration, persistently acidic urine (e.g. with chronic diarrhoea and gout) and increased oxalate absorption from the gut. In this patient, the latter is most likely given the history of extensive small bowel resection, which puts him at risk for short bowel syndrome and subsequent high oxalate reabsorption from the gut.

In the ED, the key to dealing with a patient who has suspected ureteric colic is to confirm the diagnosis and assess for complications. Confirmation of the diagnosis can be achieved through either a low-dose CT-KUB (kidneys, ureters and bladder) or ultrasound of the urinary tracts; while CT-KUB carries a radiation exposure risk, it has a much higher sensitivity than ultrasound and is generally the test of choice. Ultrasound should be used in pregnant women and is a good method of identifying hydronephrosis, but may miss small stones. The complications of kidney stones include urinary tract obstruction and infection, and therefore, renal function and urinalysis should always be checked.

The two main aspects of managing nephrolithiasis in the ED are achieving adequate pain control and predicting/facilitating stone passage. NSAIDs (e.g. rectal diclofenac, naproxen) are generally preferred for analgesia as they may decrease ureteric smooth muscle tone thereby also facilitating stone passage. With regard to stone passage, size and location are the key determinants of whether a stone is likely to pass spontaneously, with the majority of stones ≤5 mm likely to pass of their own accord. Conversely most stones ≥10 mm and/or in the proximal ureter are unlikely to pass spontaneously. Medical expulsive therapy, in the form of alpha-antagonists (e.g. tamsulosin) or calcium channel blockers (e.g. nifedipine), can be used in patients with smaller stones as there is some evidence that they help facilitate passage.

Any patient with a kidney stone in whom there is concurrent urosepsis, acute kidney injury or unyielding pain should be referred to urology for admission and consideration of intervention (antibiotics, fluids, stenting, stone retrieval, lithotripsy). However, if pain is adequately controlled and the stone is ≤5 mm, the patient may be discharged with follow-up in stone clinic. Discuss patients with stones >5 mm with the urology team who will usually arrange for the patient to come to the clinic for consideration of shockwave lithotripsy or stenting depending on the stone location. You should give safety netting advice that should the pain be unremitting, or if the patient becomes unwell (fever, vomiting, unable to pass urine), they should return to the ED for reassessment and treatment.

Key Points

- Unilateral flank pain that radiates towards the front or down towards the groin is characteristic of renal colic.
- CT-KUB is more sensitive than an ultrasound at picking up kidney stones but carries the downside of radiation exposure.
- The majority of kidney stones ≤5 mm are likely to pass spontaneously, whereas most stones >10 mm will not.

History

A 14-year-old male is brought into the Emergency Department with a 3-hour history of acute right-sided testicular pain associated with scrotal swelling and vomiting. He had been playing football at school prior to the pain starting. He is otherwise fit and well with no other medical problems or a history of having had surgery.

Examination

Examination of the testes is limited by severe pain and marked scrotal oedema. The right testis is high riding, with a horizontal lie and a diminished cremasteric reflex. The left testis is normal. His oxygen saturation on air is 98%, respiratory rate is 24, pulse is 103, blood pressure is 121/58 and temperature is 37.4°C

Questions

1. What is the diagnosis?
2. How would you manage this patient?
3. What are your concerns relating to this diagnosis?

DISCUSSION

This patient has acute right-sided testicular torsion. Torsion describes twisting of the spermatic cord resulting in obstruction of venous outflow with subsequent arterial occlusion, ischaemia and testicular necrosis. It is a urological emergency that requires urgent assessment and surgical exploration within 6 hours of the onset of pain for best salvage rates (>90%). Beyond 24 hours, the salvage rate is less than 10%, which can lead to infection, infertility and cosmetic deformity.

The classic history is acute testicular pain following minor trauma or exercise. It is commonly associated with nausea and vomiting, abnormal testicular lie (high riding, horizontal lie) and an absent cremasteric reflex, but these are not present in all patients. Slower onset testicular pain tends to occur in infection. The normal cremasteric reflex is elicited by stroking the medial aspect of the thigh, which results in the testis being pulled upwards by the cremaster muscle.

Torsion more commonly occurs in adolescents but in older men (>40) is associated with a high proportion of testicular malignancy, which should be ruled out. A predisposition is 'bell-clapper' testes, which occurs in around one-fifth of males. This is a congenital variation that can cause intravaginal torsion in adolescents when the spermatic cord rotates within the tunica vaginalis, due to the high attachment of the testicle to the tunica vaginalis. Neonates may also experience testicular torsion, not because of 'bell-clapper' testes, but because the gubernaculum has not secured the attachment of the tunica vaginalis to the spermatic cord.

If there is strong suspicion of testicular torsion, laboratory investigations or Doppler ultrasonography should not slow down surgical exploration due to the devastating consequences of delayed treatment. However, if there is clinical suspicion for other causes of acute testicular pain, such as epididymo-orchitis, then urinalysis, urine culture and a full blood count may be helpful. Beware that patients with testicular torsion may show pyuria in the urinalysis or leukocytosis on the full blood count. Doppler ultrasonography can evaluate blood flow to the testes if the suspicion of torsion is thought to be low enough that the patient does not require immediate surgical exploration. This decision should be made by a urologist.

When a patient is taken to a theatre, both sides of the scrotum will be explored with surgical fixation (orchidopexy) of both sides to prevent recurrence.

 Key Points

- Rapid onset excruciating unilateral scrotal pain combined with scrotal swelling, high riding and transverse lie testicle is associated with testicular torsion.
- Testicular torsion is a urological emergency that requires urgent surgical exploration – the best salvage rates are seen in surgical exploration less than 6 hours from the onset of the pain.
- If testicular torsion is suspected, do not let laboratory or ultrasound investigations slow down surgical exploration.

ENT, OPHTHALMOLOGY AND MAXILLOFACIAL SURGERY

CASE 68: RECURRENT NOSEBLEEDS IN A CHILD

History

A 6-year-old boy presents to the paediatric Emergency Department with a right-sided nosebleed. This is his fifth nosebleed in 4 weeks and it is always right sided. They usually last 10–15 minutes and resolve spontaneously or by pinching the nose. On this occasion, the bleed has lasted 45 minutes and the mother is very anxious.

There has been no trauma to the nose, and the child does not take any medications or have other medical problems. There is no history of easy bruising or a family history of bleeding disorders.

Examination

On examination, after suctioning and applications of co-phenylcaine spray, prominent vessels are seen on the right anterior septum. There is no blood in the back of the mouth. His cardiorespiratory parameters are within normal limits.

Blood investigations have not been performed.

Questions
1. What are the causes of recurrent epistaxis in children?
2. How would you manage a nose bleed?
3. What are the red flag nasal symptoms that may indicate a sinister disease process?

DISCUSSION

Epistaxis is common in children, affecting around half of children under 10 years of age. The bleeding most commonly derives from the anterior septum, known as Little's area. This is composed of an anastomosis of four arteries, namely, anterior ethmoid artery, spheno-palatine artery, greater palatine artery and the septal branch of the superior labial artery. Posterior nasal cavity bleeds contribute to 5%–10% of epistaxis. These occur in Woodruff's plexus, which is located over the posterior middle turbinate.

Recurrent epistaxis in children can be due to chronic inflammation and crusting from *Staphylococcus aureus* colonisation of the nasal vestibule and mucosa. This irritates the nose and results in nose picking (digital trauma), which worsens the problem. Recurrent upper respiratory tract infections also contribute to this cycle. Other causes of recurrent bleeds include trauma (from nose picking or foreign bodies) and bleeding disorders such as von Willebrand's disease or hereditary haemorrhagic telangiectasia, which are uncommon. Rarely teenage boys with recurrent nose bleeds may have juvenile nasopharyngeal angiofibroma (JNA). Therefore all patients with recurrent unilateral epistaxis should undergo naso-endoscopy by an ENT surgeon to rule out a sinister cause like JNA.

The history for epistaxis should elicit laterality, causative events like trauma, frequency and length of time, ease of bruising, medication use (especially anticoagulants) and family history of bleeding disorders. Examination of a nosebleed involves anterior rhinoscopy using an otoscope, which provides lighting and magnification. Always look in the back of the mouth, which may demonstrate blood clots or fresh blood from posterior epistaxis. Help from parents and/or experienced nurses should be sought with young or uncompliant children.

Red flags in the history include unilateral nasal symptoms such as epistaxis, discharge, blockage, facial pain, anosmia or otalgia. A unilateral mass like a polyp may be caused by a neoplasm (benign or malignant), which warrants further investigation and an urgent ENT referral for naso-endoscopy +/− CT scanning of the paranasal sinuses.

Patients with first ever nose bleeds do not require routine full blood count or coagulation screen blood tests as they do not usually provide any useful diagnostic information. In the setting of recurrent epistaxis or a history of easy bruising/family history of bleeding disorders, these blood tests can be helpful and should include coagulation screening and von Willebrand disease screening (which may cause 5%–10% of recurrent paediatric epistaxis).

Epistaxis can cause airway obstruction both at the level of the nasal cavity and further down the airway due to blood clot formation. Thus, management involves assessment and resuscitation of the patient's airway, breathing and circulation. If there has been trauma, management should follow Advanced Trauma Life Support (ATLS) guidelines.

Nosebleeds are usually minor and resolve with conservative intervention, which involves applying pressure to the anterior nasal septum (soft part of the nose), leaning forward and applying an ice pack over the forehead or back of the neck. The patient should be encouraged to do this for 20 minutes before seeking medical attention. It is also useful to do this to patients in the Emergency Department while they wait to be seen.

Should simple measures fail to stop the epistaxis, the clinician should adopt a Thudicum speculum and a good headlight. This frees up the other hand to perform suctioning, endoscopy and cautery. A cotton wool pledget soaked with co-phenylcaine solution should be inserted into the nose for 5–10 minutes. This provides analgesia and vasoconstriction to reduce bleeding. Once this has been removed, cautery using a silver nitrate stick can be very effective because approximately half of children with recurrent epistaxis have prominent vessels in Little's area. Avoid bilateral cauterisation as this increases the risk of septal perforation. If the bleeding stops, the patient can be discharged with a 2-week course of neomycin/chlorhexidine (Naseptin) antiseptic ointment, which acts to reduce bacterial colonisation. To avoid further trauma to the area that was bleeding, patients should be advised to gently apply Naspetin ointment using a cotton wool bud, or place it onto the back of a spoon and sniff it into the nose and then gently massage the external nose. Using a finger to apply the ointment can cause further trauma. Beware that Naseptin is contraindicated in patients with peanut allergy.

Absorbable haemostatic agents such as Kaltostat or Surgicel may be used over bleeding areas in addition to or instead of chemical nasal cautery. These are also useful for patients with chronic intermittent nosebleeds due to bleeding disorders like hereditary haemorrhagic telangiectasia (HHT) or chemotherapy.

Failing the above with an anterior nosebleed, packing with a merocel or Rapid Rhino pack may tamponade bleeding. When placing the pack, take care to direct it along the floor of the nose towards the tragus of the ear as if inserting a nasopharyngeal airway. Secure the silk ties or the balloon port to the side so that the mouth is not obstructed. If the bleeding is posterior, packing with a Brighton's balloon or foley catheter/BIPP ribbon may be required. Seek help from a senior ED clinician or ENT specialist early in these cases. Packs are usually left in for 24 hours before removal and re-examination. Continuing bleeding may be managed by angiographic embolisation or surgical ligation of the relevant vessels (sphenopalatine, anterior and posterior ethmoid arteries).

Upon discharge, patients should be given comprehensive verbal and written advice on the prevention of rebleeds and first-aid management should they recur. Advice should include avoiding nose picking, nose blowing, strenuous exercise, heavy lifting, hot baths, hot liquids and spicy food for up to 2 weeks.

 Key Points

- Paediatric epistaxis is a common problem, usually affecting the anterior septum.
- Recurrent paediatric epistaxis may be due to *Staphylococcus aureus* colonisation of the nasal vestibule and mucosa.
- Recurrent paediatric epistaxis should be managed by resuscitating the patient's airway, breathing and circulation. Silver nitrate cautery of prominent vessels followed by a course of neomycin/chlorhexidine (Naseptin) ointment is extremely effective. Naseptin is contraindicated in peanut allergy.
- Red flags that may indicate a sinister disease process include unilateral nasal symptoms such as epistaxis, discharge, blockage, facial pain, anosmia or otalgia. These symptoms warrant referral to ENT surgery for nasa-endoscopy +/– CT scanning of the paranasal sinuses.

History

A 4-year-old child presents with right-sided otalgia, poor appetite for the last 24 hours and a fever of 39°C. The ear pain has been worsening for the last week, and is now associated with a boggy red swelling behind the ear. There are no other obvious otological symptoms such as otorrhoea. The child suffers from recurrent ear infections and has been suffering from an upper respiratory tract infection for the last week, but is otherwise fit and well. He has not had any previous operations.

Examination

Right-sided otoscopic examination demonstrates a normal external auditory canal with a bulging, red, intact tympanic membrane. The pinna is pushed outwards due to a tender, warm, fluctuant retroauricular swelling. The left ear examination is unremarkable. Examination of the nose and throat demonstrates rhinitis and mild tonsil swelling consistent with an upper respiratory tract infection. The cranial nerve examination is unremarkable.

Questions

1. What is the diagnosis?
2. What complications are you concerned about?
3. How would you manage this patient?

DISCUSSION

This patient has acute otitis media (AOM), which is complicated by mastoiditis. This is a paediatric ENT emergency, which can have immediate and long-term complications. These include extracranial complications such as hearing loss, facial nerve palsy and a Bezold (sternocleidomastoid) or Citelli (posterior belly of digastric muscle) abscess. Intracranial complications are also possible, including meningitis or intracranial abscesses.

Following a comprehensive history and examination, appropriate investigations include an ear swab for submission to microbiology, especially if there is ear discharge. Blood tests should include a full blood count, renal function, CRP and blood cultures before starting antibiotics.

In the unwell patient, imaging in the form of a contrast enhanced CT of brain and temporal bone should be performed to look for subperiosteal or intracranial abscess ideally after review by an ENT specialist. Radiological evidence of mastoiditis includes mastoid air cell opacification and breakdown of bony trabeculae. Localised bone necrosis and resorption will result in a subperiosteal abscess.

Conservative management of AOM involves keeping the ear dry and microsuction of debris or pus in the external auditory canal (to help prevent secondary otitis externa). Medical management includes analgesia and urgent IV antibiotics as per local microbiology protocol. The commonest microorganisms are *Streptococcus pneumoniae* (60%), *Streptococcus pyogenes*, *Haemophilus influenzae* and *Staphylococcus aureus,* so a third-generation cephalosporin (e.g. ceftriaxone) with good blood–brain barrier penetration is appropriate in case of intracranial complications. The patient should also be given antibiotic eardrops such as Sofradex, which contains dexamethasone, framycetin and gramicidin until culture and sensitivity result are available.

If the patient has signs of sepsis, neurological symptoms or signs, a subperiosteal abscess or intracranial collection, then the patient will likely benefit from surgical intervention in the form of a cortical mastoidectomy +/− ventilation tube insertion into the tympanic membrane. Neurosurgical input is required if the patient has an intracranial abscess and/or central venous sinus thrombosis.

 Key Points

- Acute otitis media with mastoiditis is an emergency with potentially devastating intra- and extra-cranial complications.
- Consider a contrast enhanced CT scan of the brain and temporal bone after an ENT review, especially if the patient has neurological symptoms or signs.
- Early treatment with intravenous and topical eardrop antibiotics is essential.
- Management is multidisciplinary with regular communication between ENT surgeons, paediatricians, microbiologists, radiologists and, if appropriate, neurosurgeons.

History

An 80-year-old man presents with dysphagia to solids and liquids since eating his dinner 3 hours ago. He was eating chicken and swallowed a bone. He has pain at the level of the Adam's apple in his throat. This is the second time he has had such a problem this year. His comorbidities include hypertension and diabetes mellitus. He is a lifelong smoker and drinks 30 units of alcohol per week.

Examination

He is saturating at 96% on room air, and his respiratory rate is 28, pulse is 105 bpm and blood pressure is 110/62. He is afebrile. Palpation of the neck and neck does not demonstrate focal tenderness or surgical emphysema. His oropharynx is filled with unswallowed saliva. The remainder of his ENT examination is unremarkable.

Investigations
• A lateral soft tissue neck radiograph demonstrates a radiopaque lesion just below the level of the cricopharynx, in the shape of a bone.

Questions

1. What are the concerns with this patient?
2. What is your initial management of this patient in the ED?

DISCUSSION

This patient has a chicken bone impacted in his upper oesophagus. It may be part of a food bolus. Given his age and smoking/alcohol history, and that this is the second occurrence this year, suspicion should be raised for an underlying malignancy. A history for red flag symptoms should be sought, including dysphagia, dyspnoea, dysphonia, haemoptysis, regurgitation, referred otalgia, weight loss and a family history of head and neck cancer. This will require appropriate investigation after dealing with the acute obstruction.

The focus of the clinical encounter should establish the type of foreign body (FB) as sharp (fish or chicken bone, dentures) or corrosive (battery) foreign bodies in the upper aerodigestive tract require urgent surgical removal due to the risk of perforation, sepsis and mediastinitis. Signs of perforation include severe neck or chest pain, tachycardia, tachypneoa, fever and surgical emphysema.

Ruling out that the FB is in the upper aerodigestive tract (above the larynx and cricopharynx) can be done by an ENT surgeon using bedside flexible naso-pharyngoscopy. The history and level of pain are not accurate determinants of the level of the FB in the oesophagus. The location is sometimes established using a combination of radiographic imaging of the neck, chest and abdomen. If a lateral soft tissue neck radiograph does not show an obvious radiopaque FB, then look for loss of cervical lordosis, prevertebral soft tissue swelling and surgical emphysema. If the FB is not seen on a neck radiograph, consider a PA and lateral chest radiograph or abdominal radiograph as the FB may have migrated. Beware that the FB may not be radiopaque as is the case with certain fishbones. Radiolucent fish bones include herring, salmon, trout, mackerel and pike.

If a patient has a soft food bolus (that does not contain bone on radiographic imaging), then this may pass with time. Admit the patient and keep them nil by mouth and on IV fluids. There is no evidence base, but some clinicians use 1 mg glucagon or a carbonated beverage (10%–50% success) to relax the lower oesophageal sphincter. IV Buscopan or muscle relaxants like diazepam or morphine are also trialed by some clinicians, but caution should be taken due to their adverse effects. Carefully monitor for symptoms and signs of oesophageal perforation, and if the food bolus does not pass after 12 hours, some ENT surgeons/gastroenterologists will consider intervening to extract it using rigid or flexible oesophagoscopy.

A medically managed oesophageal food bolus should be followed up with a barium swallow and, if abnormal, OGD +/– biopsy to rule out an underlying malignant cause.

Key Points
• Foreign bodies in the upper aerodigestive tract that require immediate removal include sharp or corrosive objects including button batteries.
• Foreign bodies can cause gastrointestinal perforation, which manifests as severe neck or chest pain, tachycardia, tachypneoa, fever or surgical emphysema.

History

A 78-year-old diabetic gentleman presents with severe right-sided otalgia on the background of a 3-week history of right-sided otitis externa. He also complains of purulent otorrhoea, hearing loss, vertigo and tinnitus. He uses hearing aids.

He does not have any other medical problems but uses metformin for his diabetes. He is a lifelong smoker.

Examination

An otosocope demonstrates a normal left ear. The right ear has a markedly swollen external auditory canal with debris and pus. The tympanic membrane is not visible due to the swelling. Cranial nerve examination reveals an isolated right-sided facial nerve palsy.

Questions

1. What is the diagnosis?
2. How would you manage this patient?

DISCUSSION

This patient has malignant otitis externa (MOE), also known as necrotising otitis externa. Despite the term 'malignant', this is not a cancerous process. Rather, it refers to temporal bone (skull base) osteomyelitis. This is an ENT emergency associated with serious morbidity and mortality including cranial nerve palsies. Most commonly the facial nerve is affected, but cranial nerves 9–11 can become comprised if the jugular foramen becomes involved in the infective process. Intracranial complications include meningitis, intracerebral abscess and venous sinus thrombosis.

MOE is associated with diabetes, immunosuppression (and may lead to a new diagnosis of HIV/AIDS in young people) and haematological malignancies. It is most commonly caused by *Pseudomonas aeruginosa*, an aerobic Gram-negative rod that releases exotoxins, but can also be caused by methicillin-resistant *Staphylococcus aureus* (MRSA), Proteus and Candida species.

The defining features of MOE are severe otalgia, often exceeding oral analgesics, in the older diabetic patient. Other symptoms such as hearing loss, otorrhoea, vertigo and tinnitus may also be present or neurological signs if there are any intracranial complications.

Otosocopic examination may demonstrate granulation tissue on the osteocartilaginous junction, which is pathognomonic. There may be bone exposure. Palpation of tragus or pinna traction produces severe pain. The patient may have facial cellulitis around the ear. A full cranial nerve neurological examination especially nerves VII (stylomastoid foramen) and IX–XI (jugular foramen) is essential.

Investigations should include a full blood count to look for leukocytosis, renal function, glucose and HbA1$_c$ to assess diabetic control. An ear swab for microscopy and culture should be taken ideally before antibiotics are administered.

Perform a contrast enhanced CT scan of the brain and temporal bone to assess for intracranial complications and extent of bone destruction. CT is preferred to MRI to delineate bony involvement. However, an MRI is more sensitive for intracranial complications – the earliest sign is retrocondylar fat infiltration.

Refer the patient to the ENT team for admission and inpatient intravenous antibiotics. Typically ciprofloxacin 0.3% ear drops and ceftriaxone (anti-Pseudomonal cephalosporin with good blood–brain barrier penetration) are used. Antibiotics may need to be continued for several weeks as an outpatient.

Surgery is largely reserved for local debridement or abscess drainage and may not completely remove the disease as it tends to spread along fascial planes and vasculature.

Patient education should include advice to keep the ear dry and avoid foreign body insertion. Smoking cessation will also aid wound healing as well as optimisation of diabetic control.

 Key Points

- Malignant otitis externa (skull base osteomyelitis) should be considered in all elderly diabetic patients with severe otalgia, on the background of otitis externa.
- Ensure a full otological, cranial nerve and neurological examination is conducted. Lower cranial nerve palsies, especially the facial nerve (VII), can occur.
- Topical ciprofloxacin and intravenous ceftriaxone are indicated in the acute setting.

History

A 6-year-old child presents with a 1-hour history of frank bleeding from the mouth. Twelve hours ago, the child had a similar episode of bleeding at home, which lasted 15 minutes before self-resolution. Five days ago, he underwent a tonsillectomy under general anaesthesia for recurrent acute tonsillitis. The child has also vomited twice in the last hour; the contents of the vomitus are fresh blood and blood clots. The child is otherwise fit and well, and this was his first operation. There is no family history of bleeding disorders.

Examination

There is active bleeding from the right tonsil fossa. The remainder of the ENT examination is unremarkable. His respiratory rate is 24, saturation is 97% in room air, heart rate is 110 bpm and blood pressure is 95/60.

Questions

1. How would you manage this child?
2. What complications are you worried about?

DISCUSSION

This is an airway emergency. Post-tonsillectomy bleeding (PTB) is a common but potentially serious complication occurring in around 5%–10% of patients undergoing tonsillectomy. The majority are self-limiting but around 1% require a return to theatre to stop the bleeding.

All patients must be assessed immediately and admitted for observation as a self-limiting bleed can preclude a larger bleed within 24 hours. The indications for urgent surgical intervention are active bleeding, haemodynamic instability or a known clotting abnormality.

This child requires multidisciplinary management in the resuscitation area by an ENT surgeon, senior anaesthetist, paediatrician and emergency medicine doctor.

Airway management involves sitting the child up, leaning them forward, administering high flow oxygen (through nasal cannulae if bleeding from mouth) and encouraging the child to spit out the blood (instead of swallowing) into a bowl so contents and volume can be monitored. If the child is cooperative, suction clots from the oropharynx. Keep the child in a calm environment as crying and stress may exacerbate the bleeding.

Early intravenous (or intraosseus) access is required to resuscitate the patient. Blood should be drawn for a venous blood gas, full blood count, urea and electrolytes, clotting and group and screen. Fluid boluses using crystalloid or packed red cells at a rate of 20 mL/kg bolus should be given if there are any signs of shock.

If bleeding is severe, activate the major haemorrhage protocol and discuss the case with a haemotologist. Consider tranexamic acid early.

Other helpful measures are to administer analgesia (often the child's throat is sore from the operation) and to start broad-spectrum antibiotics in case an infection of the tonsil fossa has precipitated the bleeding. If the child has swallowed blood, he or she is likely to vomit. Therefore, give antiemetics and consider nasogastric aspiration; this can be inserted when the child is under general anaesthetic.

For patients whose bleeding has spontaneously stopped, but require observation in a hospital, give them ice cubes to suck on to soothe the pain and cause vasoconstriction of the vessels in the tonsil fossa. Three percent hydrogen peroxide gargles may also be used in older patients.

 Key Points

- Post-tonsillectomy bleeding is a relatively common complication that should be treated as an airway emergency due to the possibility of obstruction.
- Haemodynamically stable children who are not bleeding can be managed conservatively with IV antibiotics, hydrogen peroxide gargles, IV fluids and sucking on ice cubes.
- Surgery to arrest bleeding is required when children are actively bleeding, haemodynamically unstable or if they have a bleeding diathesis.

CASE 73: A SWOLLEN EYELID

History

A 6-year-old child is admitted with a 3-day history of worsening right eyelid swelling. For the past week, he has had a bad cold. His mother says he has been 'very snotty and feverish'. There was no trauma or insect bites. The child denies neurological symptoms like headache, weakness or numbness. He does not have any medical comorbidities and is up to date with immunisations.

Examination

His temperature is 37.9°C, pulse is 105, blood pressure is 101/59 and respiratory rate is 20.

On the right eye, the eyelid is inflamed and erythematous. You cannot see the underlying eye. Upon opening the eyelid, eye movements are not painful or restricted. There is no chemosis, and pupillary light reaction and visual acuity are uncompromised. The left eye is normal.

Nasal examination demonstrates green nasal discharge and gross swelling of the inferior and middle turbinates. His mucosa is rhinitic. He has generalised cervical lymphadenopathy. There is no meningism, and cranial nerve and limb neurological examination is unremarkable.

Questions

1. What is the diagnosis and cause?
2. What investigations are appropriate? When would you perform a CT scan?
3. How would you manage this patient?

DISCUSSION

This patient has periobital preseptal cellulitis, secondary to acute rhinosinusitis. This is a potential sight-threatening emergency, which can have neurological complications such as meningitis, intracranial abscesses or cavernous sinus thrombosis via direct or haematogenous spread. From the outset, it requires multidisciplinary assessment and management by ENT surgeons, ophthalmologists, paediatricians, microbiologists and radiologists. Neurosurgeons have a role if there is intracranial involvement.

The ethmoid and maxillary paranasal sinuses are most commonly infected in children, whereas in adults, the fronto-ethmoidal sinus is most commonly infected.

The history should establish the following: unilateral or bilateral eye involvement, duration of symptoms, visual deterioration, colour vision and if eye movements are full or painful. It is important to ask about neurological symptoms like headache, weakness or numbness in the face or limbs. Systemic features like fever and malaise are common. The patient's comorbidities and immunisation history are important. Precipitating factors may include upper respiratory tract infections, acute sinusitis or localised trauma (e.g. insect bites, injury).

Assessment should include comprehensive ear, nose and throat, head and neck examination as well as the cranial nerves and both eyes. Ocular exam should note chemosis, proptosis, diplopia, ophthalmoplegia, nystagmus, visual acuity and pupillary reaction. Colour vision should be tested using Ishihara plates or Hardy Rand Rittler colour vision test; loss of colour vision is one of the earliest signs of orbital complications, and must be regularly tested and clearly documented. If the patient's condition deteriorates, surgical intervention may be required to manage subperiosteal abscess, intraorbital abscess and cavernous sinus thrombosis.

Take blood for venous blood gas, full blood count, electrolytes and blood cultures. A nose swab for microbiological analysis and culture is also important.

CT scanning may be used in severe peri-orbital cellulitis or if intracranial or orbital complications are suspected. Indications include

- Visual compromise
- Proptosis
- Limited eye movement (ophthalmoplegia) or presence of binocular diplopia
- Cannot assess eye due to eyelid swelling
- No clinical improvement after 24–48 hours medical therapy evidenced by persistent fever, worsening inflammatory markers

Early administration of broad-spectrum intravenous antibiotics such as co-amoxyclav or ceftriaxone is crucial. Follow local microbiology guidelines to cover the commonest micro-organisms, namely *Staphylococcus aureus*, *Staphylococcus epidermis*, *Streptococcus pneumoniae*, *Streptococus pyogenes*, *Moraxella catarhallis* and anaerobes. *Haemophilus influenzae* is less common since the introduction of the HIB vaccination.

To reduce the inflammatory process and allow paranasal sinus drainage, administer corticosteroid drops such as Betnesol® (betamethasone 0.1% and neomycin 0.5%) and nasal decongestants such as paediatric Otrivine® (xylometalazone hydrochloride 0.05%). If there are any signs of visual compromise, consider oral steroids.

Have a low threshold for admission in these patients as the cellulitis can often spread rapidly. When a patient is discharged, ensure they have triple therapy, namely antibiotics, nasal decongestants and nasal steroids. The patient or parent should be counseled on the correct technique for administering nasal drops (in the head down position, or head extension off the edge of a bed). Also, ensure they have early follow-up with an ophthalmologist. They should return if there is any deterioration in vision (especially colour), painful eye movements, failure to improve or any neurological symptoms or signs.

🔑 **Key Points**

- Periorbital cellulitis is a potentially sight-threatening emergency. It is often precipitated by an upper respiratory tract infection, rhinosinusitis or local trauma (injury, insect bite).
- Investigations should include a nose swab for microbiology and contrast-enhanced CT scan of paranasal sinuses and the brain if there is visual compromise, reduced acuity, proptosis or ophthalmoplgia, or if the eye cannot be assessed due to severe swelling.
- Treatment includes treating rhinosinusitis as well as the periorbital abscess. This includes intranasal steroids, decongestants and saline douching and intravenous antibiotics.
- Joint care among ENT surgeons, ophthalmologists and paediatricians is recommended.

History

A 38-year-old car mechanic attends the Emergency Department with a 1-day history of progressive pain in his right eye. He remembers angle-grinding a piece of exhaust at work without any eye protection. He found it very difficult to sleep and is concerned that there is something in his eye. The pain appears to be better in a dark environment and if he keeps his eyes closed.

Examination

Physical examination is difficult to perform, as the patient is reluctant to open his right eye under usual room lighting. Visual acuity is 6/6 in the left eye, and 6/12 that improves to 6/6 with pinhole in the right eye. The pupillary reflex is normal with no relative apparent pupillary defect (RAPD). Slit lamp examination shows an injected conjunctiva with an increased marginal tear film. There is a 1 mm reflective metallic flake with a brown halo on the cornea at the 6 o-clock position.

Questions

1. Which metallic corneal foreign bodies are of particular concern?
2. How would you remove the corneal foreign body?
3. What further management is required?

DISCUSSION

This patient has a corneal foreign body. Any patient reporting sharp pain with photosensitivity, watery discharge and foreign body sensation should prompt the emergency physician to review the ocular surface.

Start your examination by documenting visual acuity – the patient may require topical anaesthesia (oxybuprocaine, tetracaine, proxymetacaine, lidocaine) to assist with this. Slit lamp examination of the eye should involve a systematic review of the upper and lower external eyelid, the conjunctiva and cornea. Findings should be drawn accurately on patient records for comparison at a later date. Remember to perform tarsal eversion to look for trapped foreign bodies and/or perform a sweep of the conjunctival fornices of the affected eye with a topical anaesthetic soaked cotton bud tip.

The anterior chamber should be assessed for depth and evidence of inflammation and the pupil assessed for shape and reactivity. Assessing anterior chamber inflammation can be difficult to assess. One method that can be used is to first focus the slit beam onto the pupil margin and then slightly pull back on the slit lamp to defocus, thereby focusing into the anterior chamber. Slit beam should be on highest brightness and set to a 1 mm by 1 mm box to identify cellular activity in the anterior chamber. This may resemble a starry cosmos. Depth of anterior chamber is difficult to gauge without having the experience of examining several eyes. One gross method is to ensure there is a general separation between iris and cornea. A more refined yet useful method for assessing angle closure was described by Van Herick. This involves angling the slit beam 60 degrees near the limbus; the resultant effect causes the light beam to hit the cornea and cast a shadowing beam on the iris. The ratio of the space between the light reflected on the cornea and iris is grossly related to the depth of the angle. A 1:1 thickness of the empty space and the thickness of the corneal reflection suggests open angles; a 1:4 or small ratio may suggest angle closure.

Abnormal pupil shape, iris defect and shallow anterior chamber are red flags for possible ocular perforation or penetrating ocular injury. Should you suspect an anterior chamber leak, you can assess for this by instilling a drop of fluorescein. This will stain the tear film and an aqueous leak may be evident. This is known as the Seidel test. Fluorescein may also cause corneal foreign bodies to be highlighted by a ring of dye.

However, most metal foreign bodies are usually obvious as they reflect the slit lamp beam and will typically glisten on the cornea. Certain metals will also react with the corneal tissue and cause rust rings as in this case. Table 74.1 highlights metal types and their relative reactivity.

Most conjunctival foreign bodies can be removed by simply irrigating the eye or by using a cotton bud tip soaked in topical anaesthetic.

Removing a corneal foreign body, as in this case, requires more skill and an experienced operator should be sought. Peripheral lesions can be removed without any major consequences to the patient. Centrally located foreign bodies should be approached with caution.

Table 74.1 **Materials and ocular reactivity**

Reactivity	Material
Inert	Carbon, gold, silver, coal, stone, glass, plastic
Mild	Nickel, aluminum, mercury, zinc
Severe	Iron, steel, copper, wood

To remove a corneal surface foreign body, first apply topical anaesthesia to the affected eye, and inform the patient of possible deterioration of symptoms when the anaesthesia wears off. Ask the patient to look straight ahead and visualise the target on the slit-lamp. This allows for good magnification and illumination, but also prevents the patient from moving. Hold the eyelid to prevent blinking. Then, gently tease the material off the corneal surface with the tip of an 18–25 gauge needle. A successful removal will involve creating a surgical corneal abrasion, which will generally heal rapidly.

Should there be a residual rust ring, refer this to the local ophthalmology service for removal with a burr tool. The eye will need topical antibiotic ointment or drops and oral analgesics, and some patients find patching of the eye provides symptomatic relief. Remember to ask about tetanus status and assess for immunoglobulin or booster if vaccination status is unclear.

In uncomplicated cases without rust ring and complete removal off the visual axis, the patient may be discharged without routine follow-up. Larger abrasions or those on the visual axis should be referred for routine review in clinic at 48–72 hours with advice to attend earlier if there are problems. Large defects >2 mm, central defects or patients with rust rings should be reviewed within 24 hours.

Embedded foreign bodies or penetrating trauma should be referred for immediate review for wound exploration and closure under general anaesthesia.

 Key Points

- Pain with photosensitivity, watery discharge and foreign body sensation are cardinal features of corneal irritation.
- Visual acuity should be documented in all patients presenting with any visual symptoms.
- The Seidel test is a useful test to exclude penetrating ocular trauma, which is an ophthalmic emergency.
- Iron, steel, copper and wood are known to cause severe ocular reactions and should be removed completely from the ocular surface prior to discharge.

CASE 75: PAINFUL RED EYE

History

A 28-year-old woman attends the Emergency Department with a 12-hour history of moderate gritty right eye pain, which is worse in bright lighting conditions, and a clear watery discharge. She denies any flashes, floaters, glare or history of trauma to that eye. She is a regular contact lens wearer using monthly soft lenses. She tells you that she sometimes forgets to remove the lenses and sleeps with them in. There is no other past medical or ocular history of note.

Examination

Vital signs are normal. Right eye visual acuity is slightly reduced (6/9) compared to the left eye (6/6). Physical examination demonstrates intentional squinting of her right eye. The conjunctiva is diffusely injected and the cornea is hazy on inspection. On slit-lamp examination, there is 1 mm fluorescein uptake para-central at the 9 o'clock position.

Questions

1. What is your differential diagnosis?
2. What are the key risk factors for the most likely diagnosis presented here?
3. What investigations are required?
4. How would you manage this patient?

DISCUSSION

Painful red eye is a concerning sign for emergency physicians; however, clues in history and examination help differentiate benign and sight threatening ophthalmic emergencies (see Table 75.1).

The history and examination findings in this patient are suggestive of microbial keratitis, which is an ophthalmological emergency. This may be viral, bacterial, fungal or protozoal. In this case, bacterial keratitis is suspected as the patient admits to poor hygiene with lens wearing and has a non-dendritic, punctate ulcer; however, one must also consider *Acanthamoeba* in the differential diagnosis.

The following risk factors should raise suspicion of this potentially sight-threatening condition and should be evaluated in your history:

- Epithelial defects – existing abrasions and non-healing epithelial defects.
- Frequent contact lens wear – poor hygiene and extended wear carry a greater risk.
- Pre-existing ocular surface disease or conditions that may exacerbate this such as lid malposition or long-term use of preservative containing eye drops or steroids.
- Previous corneal surgery.
- Systemic immunodeficiency, diabetes, rheumatoid arthritis and vitamin A deficiency.

In terms of other differentials, glaucoma is unlikely as the patient is young, is not diabetic and does not have uncontrolled hypertension. There is no history of systemic or rheumatic disease that may suggest an associated episcleritis or scleritis, and there is no history of direct trauma. A simple conjunctivitis or corneal abrasion is possible, but the crucial finding is a punctate corneal staining on fluorescein staining suggestive of an infiltrative pathology.

Initial management of *bacterial* keratitis should include removing contact lenses from both eyes. Lesions require corneal scrapes for microscopy, culture and sensitivity prior to antimicrobial treatment. Initial treatment involves topical antimicrobial therapy, commonly a fluoroquinolone (e.g. ciprofloxacin or levofloxacin), every 1–2 hours for the initial 24–48 hours. This is usually sufficient to sterilise the corneal surface; subsequently, the frequency may be reduced to minimise the side effects from topical quinolones. Oral antibiotics may be considered for patients with deep ulcers or scleral involvement.

Corneal scrapes are normally performed by an ophthalmologist or trained healthcare professional under topical anaesthesia (e.g. tetracaine 1% topical preparation). Using a slit-lamp,

Table 75.1 **Common causes of red eye**

Eyelids and orbit	Conjunctival	Corneal	Other
Blepharitis	Conjunctivitis	Pterygium	Trauma
Trichiasis	• Infectious	Foreign body	Ocular surface
Malposition	• Allergic	Chemical burn	disease
Lagophthalmos	• Chemical	Abrasion	Endophthalmitis
Acne rosacea	Pingeculitis	Keratitis	Anterior uveitis
Dacryocystitis,	Subconjunctival	• Bacterial	Angle closure
canuliculitis	haemorrhage	• Fungal	glaucoma
Orbital cellulitis	Symblepharon	• *Acanthomoeba*	Episcleritis
	Rare cases,	• Viral (HSV, VZV)	Scleritis
	neoplasias	Contact lens associated	
		keratopathy	

a 25G needle is used to slide across the surface of the lesion ideally capturing the base and edge of the ulcer. The material collected should be then transferred to a culture plate without breaking the medium. Routine plates include blood agar (bacterial), chocolate agar (bacterial), Sabouraud-dextrose agar (fungal) and glass plates for Gram staining. In patients that you suspect have fungal keratitis (satellite lesions, feathery edges, history of vegetative trauma), it is important to discuss this with the microbiologist so appropriate length of culture and slide stains can be applied.

Acanthamoeba keratitis is a rare, sight-threatening condition. It is a protozoan that is abundant in fresh water, and contact lens wearers with poor hygiene such as washing lenses in tap water and wearing lenses in the shower are at increased risk. Clinically, patient may report severe pain that is not proportional to signs observed, which may resemble viral keratitis; This, care should be given examination may reveal similarities to viral keratitis; thus, care should be given to diagnosing HSV keratitis in contact lens wearers. Microbiological diagnosis may be made with corneal scrapes, PCR and confocal microscopy, the latter being available in very few specialized centres.

Prognosis is good if caught early, but complications including corneal perforation and corneal scarring may occur. The mainstay of treatment is mainly medical, but corneal grafting or transplant may be required.

Patients will need regular follow-up with the ophthalmologist until improvement is seen. Infections can be difficult to treat and recurrence is common in fungal or protozoan infections.

Hygiene and education about safe lens wearing is paramount, and the patient should be counseled regarding this once the acute infection has cleared.

 Key Points

- In patients with red eyes, reduced vision with severe to moderate pain should be prompted to an early ophthalmology review.
- Pre-existing ocular surface disease and contact lens wear are high risk factors for microbial keratitis.
- In patients who wear contact lenses, severe pain and a corneal ulcer suggest *Acanthamoeba* keratitis.

History

A 29-year-old male is brought to the Emergency Department after an alleged assault with a table leg. He reports increasing pain and deterioration in vision in the left eye. This is associated with a mild headache, but he denies any nausea, vomiting or blackouts. He has a history of asthma managed with inhaled salbutamol. He has no past ophthalmic history.

Examination

Vital signs: temperature of 35.8°C, blood pressure of 140/80, heart rate of 90 and regular, respiratory rate of 30, 100% O_2 saturations on air.

The patient is alert and oriented. He has marked swelling around the orbit and the left globe appears proptosed but intact. He has diplopia in all positions and eye movements are reduced. His visual acuity in the right eye is 6/6 but is reduced to counting fingers in the left eye.

Investigations
• The Seidel test is negative.

Questions

1. What is the significance of the Seidel test?
2. What further investigations are required?
3. What immediate management is required? Describe the subsequent management of this patient.

DISCUSSION

Thirty percent of all facial fractures involve the orbit, of which the majority affect the orbital floor, also referred to as a 'blowout' fracture. The relatively thicker lateral and superior orbital rim provides firm support and protection, creating a weakness in the orbital floor, thus saving the globe from rupture.

Due to the serious nature of the mechanisms that result in orbital injuries, one must first exclude any neurologic injuries, which are prioritised over ocular injuries. Assess the patient in accordance to ATLS guidelines including full assessment of the cervical spine. Should there be suspicion of spinal injury, immobilise the patient and image the spine to exclude injury. There has been a move towards CT in most centres, and it provides an opportunity to scan the head, orbits, facial bones and cervical spine concurrently.

After intracranial and cervical spine injuries have been excluded, progress to a detailed ophthalmic assessment. Examination should assess visual acuity and colour vision, which reflect visual prognosis. Further examination should include globe position, eye movement, sensory examination of the supra- and infra-orbital nerve distribution, presence of a relative afferent pupillary defect (RAPD) and careful palpation of the orbital rim to note any step deformity. In open globe injuries with visible penetrating objects, it may be tempting to remove the object; however, avoid this as it may cause the globe to collapse.

The Seidel test is useful in the traumatic setting, especially to establish any occult open globe injuries. The test is conducted by instilling fluorescein onto the ocular surface. Using a cobalt-blue light from a slit lamp, the aim is to see whether there is any aqueous humour leakage washing the fluorescein away – a waterfall appearance on a background of green fluorescein. In such cases, the test is considered positive and a sign of open globe injury. A negative Seidel test with a soft globe (malformed eye, collapsed cornea, intra-ocular pressure <10 mmHg) with conjunctival folding should raise suspicion of posterior globe rupture and be referred to an ophthalmologist urgently.

Royal College of Radiology guidelines state facial x-rays remain the first initial investigation in facial trauma and can help identify most foreign bodies. However, if trauma head scans are being performed, concurrent HRCT of the orbits with 1 mm axial sections and coronal reconstruction provide an excellent modality to assess for fractures, foreign body and globe integrity. Alternatively, an MRI provides excellent soft tissue differentiation and is therefore useful in determining secondary neurologic damage or wooden foreign bodies. Metallic ferrous-containing foreign bodies must be fully excluded prior to considering an MRI.

The case presented highlights the cardinal signs of ocular compartment syndrome caused by retrobulbar haemorrhage – proptosis, restriction of eye movement, RAPD, reduced visual acuity, colour vision and worsening pain. Delay in recognition and treatment can result in permanent visual loss.

Lateral cantholysis (canthotomy) is an emergency measure that can relieve compartment syndrome and buy time for definitive treatment. There is low risk of morbidity associated with the procedure, so if in doubt, it is better to perform the procedure than risk preventable visual loss. In case of a retrobulbar haemorrhage, a lateral cantholysis will allow time for haemostasis and resorption of blood. Lateral cantholysis is not suitable in certain patient groups (e.g. those with a bleeding risk or on anticoagulation), and such individuals can be medically managed with intravenous mannitol solution, high-dose steroids and anti-glaucomatous drops.

Uncomplicated orbital fractures (e.g. orbital blowout without rectus entrapment, not involving the globe) in stable patients should be referred to the maxillofacial team and ophthalmology, the latter to exclude occult globe injury. Patients should be advised to sleep upright and avoid blowing the nose, excessive coughing or bending, all of which may worsen the condition for the next 4–6 weeks. In cases of severe dysmotility, a short course of steroids (0.5–1.0 mg/kg) can be used to reduce localised oedema. The use of broad spectrum antibiotics (co-amoxiclav) is debatable, and therefore local policy should be followed.

Key Points

- Orbital trauma is often associated with polytrauma, affecting young males.
- The Seidel test can help identify occult anterior open globe injuries. However, it can be negative in posterior scleral rupture.
- CT of the orbit with 1 mm slices is a sensitive and specific investigation in suspected intra-ocular injuries, and is useful for planning orbital reconstruction.
- Early recognition and management of orbital compartment syndrome with lateral cantholysis is required to prevent permanent visual loss.

History

An 18-year-old man attends the Emergency Department after falling off his bicycle. He stopped suddenly when a pedestrian crossed, forcing him to press the handbrakes and was thrown forward. He landed on his arm and hit his jaw. He got up immediately; however, the jaw pain has worsened to the point whereby he can no longer open his mouth.

Examination

Vital signs are normal and he has no cervical spine tenderness. Examination of the face reveals a graze on the chin and maximal jaw opening of 30 degrees. He has bilateral symmetrical step deformities adjacent to the chin and some maxillary tenderness. He also has reduced sensation of his lower lip. His occlusion is misaligned; however, he has no loose teeth.

Questions

1. What initial investigations would you perform?
2. How would you manage this patient?
3. What advice would you give to this patient?

DISCUSSION

Facial injuries can range in severity from life-threatening to simple lacerations. They are often associated with other potentially serious multi-system trauma, and, as such, trauma patients should be assessed and managed as per ATLS guidelines including careful assessment of head, neck and potential airway injury.

Understanding the mechanism can help predict common fracture patterns (Table 77.1). Common fracture patterns that can be seen involve the parasymphysis. Bilateral parasymphyseal fractures can result in a bucket-handle fracture, which can result in airway compromise due to loss of support to the tongue. Other common fractures are angle and condylar fracture (the latter can occur in isolation). In the elderly, a fall or fainting can result in classic bilateral condylar fractures with a midline or para-midline fracture of the mandible, referred to as guardsman fracture. Furthermore, understanding the location of the injury to anatomy may help predict recovery; for example, injuries that occur to the lateral aspect of the jaw may fracture along the mandibular canal, which contains the inferior alveolar neurovascular bundle.

Jaw pain, altered bite, numbness of lower lip, trismus or difficulty moving the jaw are the cardinal symptoms of possible mandible fracture or dislocation. On clinical examination, a pathognomonic feature is altered occlusion and/or presence of sublingual haematoma. The patient's jaw line should be palpated for any gross step deformity; alternatively, gently apply pressure to the patient's chin. The latter is a crude clinical test to determine the integrity of the jaw, which should withstand small forces comfortably.

If a mandibular fracture is suspected, plain radiological imaging is the initial test of choice – orthopantomogram (OPG) and postero-anterior (PA) views should be performed. Alternatively, plain x-rays taken 90 degrees to each other might be sufficient to diagnose fracture. In cases with multisystem involvement, a CT scan of the head with facial views and 3D reconstruction is also diagnostic. When assessing radiographs of the mandible, it is important to appreciate that the structure of the mandible should be considered as a ring. Thus, if you note one fracture line, look for another.

As mentioned above, all facial injuries should be assessed based on the ATLS principles. Adequate analgesia will make the examination easier to perform. Ensure that the patient's tetanus vaccination is up-to-date, and administer prophylactic antibiotics (e.g. co-amoxiclav) as most mandible fractures are considered to be open injuries. Patients should be informed

Table 77.1 **Common mechanism of injury and anatomic site of fracture**

Mandible site	Assault (%)	Road traffic accident (%)	Fall (%)
Angle	25	10	10
Body	25	10	25
Ramus	10	7	1
Subcondyle/ Condyle	20	25	30
Symphasis/ Parasymphsis	20	45	30
Alveolus	0	3	4

to start a soft diet to maintain nutrition but minimise pain and mandible misalignment. Wounds should also be assessed and basic wound care should be given.

The patient should be referred to the local oral and maxillofacial surgery team for further management. This may include temporary fixation (inter-maxillary fixation devices) in the emergency setting to stabilise the mandible, but also can be the management of choice for stable, closed fractures. Alternatively, patients may require open reduction and internal fixation of the mandible in displaced or complex fractures.

 Key Points

- Facial injuries can range from simple to life-threatening/changing injuries.
- All facial trauma should be assessed in line with ATLS principles.
- Mandibular fractures may have more than one fracture point. However, condylar fractures can be isolated.
- Loss of genioglossus support can result in airway comprise and requires early maxillofacial surgery input and anaesthetic.

PAEDIATRICS

CASE 78: COUGH AND DIFFICULTY BREATHING IN AN INFANT

History

A 3-month-old male presents to the Emergency Department with a 3-day history of cough and coryza. His breathing has become more laboured, and he has reduced fluid intake. His nappies are less wet than usual.

He was born by spontaneous vaginal delivery at 35+2 weeks gestation and required continuous positive airway pressure due to respiratory distress. He was treated with intravenous antibiotics for suspected sepsis; however, cultures were negative. There were no antenatal concerns. He has been well since. He has an older sister who attends nursery and has also recently had similar coryzal symptoms.

Examination

Vital signs: respiratory rate of 70–80 breaths/minute, heart rate of 180 beats/minute, O_2 saturation of 96% on room air, apyrexial.

He is actively coughing and has subcostal and intercostal recessions. Auscultation demonstrates crackles and wheezing throughout the chest. His heart sounds are normal. He is 'pink' with palpable femoral pulses and a central capillary return of 3 seconds. The rest of the examination is unremarkable.

Questions

1. What is the diagnosis?
2. What further investigations must be performed in the Emergency Department?
3. Outline the key principles in treating this patient.

DISCUSSION

This patient has a clinical picture suggestive of a diagnosis of bronchiolitis. This is an acute respiratory condition, often caused by a viral infection, resulting in inflammation of the bronchioles. The effects of this include increased mucus secretion, bronchial narrowing and obstruction. This may lead to air trapping, atelectasis, alveolar injury and reduced ventilation leading to a ventilation–perfusion mismatch.

Bronchiolitis occurs in children under 2 years of age and most commonly presents in infants aged 3 to 6 months. It most frequently occurs in association with viral infections such as respiratory syncytial virus (RSV) in around 75% of cases and is most prevalent in the winter and spring months.

Children most at risk of severe bronchiolitis include those with chronic lung disease, congenital heart disease, premature birth (particularly under 32 weeks), neuromuscular disorders, immunodeficiency and those aged less than 3 months at presentation.

Symptoms of bronchiolitis in children include breathing difficulties, cough, poor feeding, irritability and, in the very young, apnoea. Signs may include wheezing and/or crepitations on auscultation and mild pyrexia. Symptoms usually peak between days 3 and 5 of the illness.

Do not routinely perform blood tests/gases or chest radiographs in children with bronchiolitis unless you suspect another diagnosis or the patient is deteriorating. Rapid virological PCR testing is recommended if admitting the patient. This helps with cohorting patients with the same virus strains into the same bay on the ward.

The mainstay of treatment is supportive care. Consider upper airway suctioning in patients with secretions and associated respiratory distress or feeding difficulties. Oxygen supplementation is required if saturations persistently fall below 92% in air.

The child may need high flow oxygen therapy (e.g. Optiflow) or continuous positive airway pressure (CPAP) if there are signs of worsening respiratory failure. Commence fluids by nasogastric or orogastric tube if the child cannot take sufficient amounts orally, and consider intravenous fluids if they cannot tolerate this or if they have impending respiratory failure.

Signs of impending respiratory failure include exhaustion (laboured breathing), recurrent apnoea or failure to maintain adequate oxygen saturations despite oxygen supplementation.

Around 3% of all infants under 1 year old are admitted to hospital with bronchiolitis. Indications for admission include observed or reported apnoea, oxygen saturation less than 92% in air, insufficient fluid intake (less than 50%–75% of normal intake in past 24 hours) or persisting severe respiratory distress.

 Key Points

- Bronchiolitis is predominantly caused by respiratory syncytial virus (RSV).
- Although bronchiolitis is a clinical diagnosis, rapid virological PCR testing is helpful for cohorting patients on the ward.
- Not all patients require hospital admission. Hospital admission is required for supportive therapy when patients require supplementary oxygen or fluid therapy, and those with signs of pending respiratory failure.

History

A 15-month-old female presents to the Emergency Department with a 1 day history of coryza, a 'barking' cough and 'funny breathing noises'. She has been off solid food today and fluid intake is slightly reduced; however, she is continuing to wet her nappies as normal.

She had a normal birth history. She has no significant medical history and immunisations are up to date. Developmentally, she is in keeping with her peers.

Examination

Temperature of 37.7°C, respiratory rate of 45–50 breaths/minute, heart rate of 120–130 beats/minute.

She is alert, pink and well perfused, and smiles appropriately with parents. She has stridor and good air entry bilaterally in her chest. She does, however, have moderate subcostal and intercostal recessions with normal heart sounds. The rest of the examination is unremarkable.

Questions

1. What is the diagnosis?
2. What investigations should be performed in the Emergency Department?
3. What is the management of this condition?

DISCUSSION

This patient has a clinical diagnosis of croup or laryngotracheitis.

This is a respiratory illness of the upper airway characterised by inspiratory stridor, barking cough and hoarseness. These symptoms occur as a result of oedema of the larynx and trachea, which has been triggered by a recent viral infection, usually Parainfluenza virus. It typically occurs in children aged 6 months to 3 years of age. More severe croup can be associated with respiratory distress, cyanosis and upper airway obstruction.

It is important to consider differential diagnoses of upper airway obstruction on assessment, for example:

1. *Epiglottitis* – Drooling, agitated child who does not usually have a cough.
2. *Bacterial tracheitis* – Toxic-looking child with a barking cough and stridor with high fever, and has not responded to treatment for croup.
3. *Inhaled foreign body* – Sudden onset of stridor in a well child.
4. *Anaphylaxis* – Associated swelling of the face and tongue, often with urticaria and wheezing.

It is important to avoid upsetting the child on assessment as this could exacerbate the stridor; therefore, it is usually advised to leave the child with the parent in a comfortable position, and to avoid inserting tongue depressors or intravenous cannulas, or taking chest radiographs.

Management of croup includes adequate fluid hydration and oral steroids (dexamethasone), which help to reduce airway oedema. If the child cannot tolerate oral intake, consider nebulised steroids such as budesonide. The child may improve with this therapy and can be discharged after a period of observation. If discharging these patients, as dexamethasone has a short half-life, they may require a second dose 12 hours later. They should be warned to return to the hospital if they develop stridor or experience worsening difficulty in breathing.

In severe croup, enlist senior help from paediatricians and anaesthetists as the child may require intubation and transfer to the Paediatric ICU (PICU). Nebulised adrenaline (0.5 mL/kg of 1:1000 solution up to a maximum of 5 mL) along with nebulised budesonide (2 mg) should be given as first line. This may reduce upper airway oedema and allow for improvement. A further dose may be administered as necessary upon senior advice and high-dose dexamethasone (600 mcg/kg) should be given.

These patients might require urgent intubation and seek early support from paediatric anaesthetists and your local PICU retrieval team. Also, be prepared for a difficult intubation with a range of endotracheal tube sizes and the difficult airway trolley.

 Key Points

- Croup, or laryngotracheitis, is a respiratory illness of the upper airway characterised by inspiratory stridor, barking cough and hoarseness.
- It usually resolves with oral steroids and hydration, but in severe cases may require nebulised adrenaline, higher dose steroids and intubation with monitoring in PICU.

History

A 4-month-old female presents with pyrexia. Her mother informs you that she has 'not been herself today'. She has had reduced fluid intake but continues to wet her nappies. She has been pyrexial for the last 3 days, with the highest recorded temperature being 39.4°C at home today. There are no other associated symptoms. She had a normal birth history and has no significant medical history. She is due to have her third set of immunisations next week. Her older brother has recently been at home with a 'chest infection'.

Examination

Her temperature is 39.6°C. She has a capillary refill time of 4 seconds centrally and 3 seconds peripherally, with a heart rate of 170 beats/minute. Blood pressure is within normal limits. The infant appears miserable and is crying inconsolably. She has dry mucous membranes but palpable femoral pulses. The rest of your examination is unremarkable with no obvious focus for infection.

Questions

1. Which investigations should be performed in the Emergency Department?
2. Outline the key principles in managing feverish illnesses in children.

DISCUSSION

This child has pyrexia of unknown origin. She should be adequately assessed in the Emergency Department and managed accordingly.

Fever is a very common presentation in the Emergency Department, and in the immuno-competent child is usually caused by a simple infection (usually viral or bacterial) with common sources being the chest, urine, ear, nose or throat. Diagnosis is mostly based on clinical history and examination, but in some cases, no obvious focus can be identified.

Other causes of fever may include less common infections such as parasitic infections, malignancy such as solid tumours and leukaemia, vascular and autoimmune diseases such as juvenile arthritis and Kawasaki disease and other conditions such as Familial Mediterranean Fever.

On assessment, it is important to look for concerning features. Tachycardia is a particular feature that should not be ignored, especially if the patient remains tachycardic after the use of anti-pyretics. This immediately places the child in a higher-risk group for serious illness.

The following clinical features are also red-flag signs for serious illness:

- Grunting, tachypneoa or other signs of respiratory distress
- Mottled, pale skin with cool peripheries and prolonged capillary refill time
- Irritability, with a high-pitched cry, and if the child is not responding to social cues
- Difficulty to rouse or a bulging fontanelle
- An 'ill'-looking child

In the above case, no obvious source of infection was found on examination. The patient should be considered for a septic screen including blood tests (capillary blood gas, full blood count, renal function, liver function, C-reactive protein and blood cultures), urinalysis and culture. A chest radiograph is recommended if the white cell count is >20 × 10⁹/L. A lumbar puncture should also be considered to exclude meningitis if no immediate source is found as per current NICE guidelines for children under 1 year of age.

Children with pyrexia of unknown origin should be referred to the paediatric team for admission, observation and further investigation and treatment as necessary. Pitfalls in the ED include the failure to realise the severity of illness in the early stages (capillary blood gas testing is a quick way to assess for severe metabolic insult).

After taking the relevant cultures for microbiolical analysis, the use of early parenteral antibiotic treatment should be considered in unwell or toxic children, and most hospitals will have specific antibiotic protocols for empiric treatment stratified by age. Fluid resuscitation should also be quickly administered if there are concerns about sepsis and haemodynamic compromise.

🔑	Key Points

- Infants <1 month of age presenting with fever >38°C will need a full septic screen, as per NICE guidelines.
- A thorough history and clinical examination is key to determining causes of fever. Do not forget less common sites of infection, such as a septic joint.
- A recent travel history may provide valuable information if no obvious source is immediately identified.
- Consider Kawasaki disease in fever lasting more than 5 days.
- If no source is found, refer to the paediatric team for admission and further investigation.
- In the unwell child, do not delay the administration of empirical parenteral broad spectrum antibiotics and fluid resuscitation.

History

A 2-year-old male presents to the Emergency Department with a 2-day history of diarrhoea and vomiting. The symptoms are worsening in frequency. He has only managed to tolerate half of his fluid intake today without vomiting, and has had at least four episodes of loose, watery stool with reduced urine output. There is no blood or mucous in the stool. He is 'not himself'. He has not had any recent travel abroad, although his father is at home with similar symptoms. The patient does not have a significant birth or medical history. Immunisations are up to date.

Examination

His cardiorespiratory observations and temperature are normal.

The patient appears miserable. He has warm peripheries but slightly dry mucous membranes. Capillary refill time is 3 seconds centrally and 3 seconds peripherally. He has good volume peripheral pulses. His abdominal examination is normal.

Questions

1. What is the most likely diagnosis and its underlying pathophysiology?
2. What further assessment and investigations must be performed in the Emergency Department?
3. Outline the key principles in treating this patient.

DISCUSSION

This child has a clinical picture suggestive of gastroenteritis.

Gastroenteritis is a very common condition causing inflammation of the gastrointestinal tract. Clinical features are secondary to infection and destruction of enterocytes. This results in transudation of fluid into the intestinal lumen and loss of fluid and salt in the stool. In addition, this decreases the ability to digest and absorb food across the mucosa.

The most common cause in the child under 5 years is rotavirus. This can be easily transferred to food, objects and surfaces if strict hygiene is not practiced. It is estimated that almost every child will have at least one rotavirus infection before the age of 5, and many children will have several episodes a year.

The main symptoms are diarrhoea and vomiting, and some children may also have associated pyrexia or abdominal pain. It is important that the child is clinically assessed for the degree of dehydration in the Emergency Department. This child already has a reduced urine output and change in behaviour. His examination yields signs suggestive of mild dehydration.

Other infective causes include *Salmonella* or *E. coli* infections. Parasitic infections such as *Giardia* should be suspected after travelling abroad and typically present with very frothy diarrhoea. Stool culture can help distinguish between these pathogens but typically takes 72 hours to yield preliminary results.

Extra-intestinal infections may also present with diarrhoea and vomiting, such as meningitis, urinary tract infection and lobar pneumonia particularly in younger children.

If the symptoms are persistent, non-infectious causes of diarrhoea and vomiting may also be considered. These include bowel obstruction, inflammatory bowel disease, malabsorption disorders, food allergy and malignancy.

Blood tests are not routinely indicated but in indeterminate cases, a capillary blood gas is a useful point-of-care test to look at acid–base balance, electrolytes and glucose. Perform stool microbiological investigations if septicaemia is suspected, if there is blood/mucous in the stool or if the child is immunocompromised. This should also be considered if the child has recently been abroad, if there is uncertainty about the diagnosis or if the diarrhoea has not settled within 7 days.

The first-line treatment for clinical dehydration is oral rehydration therapy, using low osmolarity oral rehydration solution (ORS). The patient should be encouraged to have small sips often and be observed for a time period to assess the clinical response to this. This can be supplemented with their usual feeds (e.g. milk or water), but it is advised not to offer fruit juices or carbonated drinks. Consider administering the ORS via nasogastric tube if there is persistent vomiting or if the patient is unable to drink, and consider giving fluid deficit replacement and maintenance fluid via this method if clinically indicated.

Use intravenous fluid therapy if shock is suspected or confirmed and monitor for red-flag features (e.g. if the child appears unwell, altered responsiveness, sunken eyes, tachycardia, tachypneoa, reduced skin turgor). Intravenous fluids should also be used if oral fluids or nasogastric tube cannot be tolerated.

This patient was clinically assessed to have mild dehydration. If a trial of ORS was tolerated, and the patient remained clinically stable, they can be discharged home. The family should be advised to continue with ORS at home in addition to milk and water and to return if fluid intake is less than half of normal, if urine output is decreased or if the patient becomes lethargic and unwell.

🔑 | **Key Points**

- Gastroenteritis is common in children. Rotavirus is the commonest cause in children younger than 5 years.
- Assessing and treating hydration disturbances is essential.
- It is not essential to perform laboratory or stool culture investigations on all patients with diarrhoea.
- Treatment includes oral rehydration therapy, which can also be administered by NG tube in cases of severe vomiting.

History

A 2-year-old girl presents to the Emergency Department with complaints of central abdominal pain and a change in behaviour. She has been urinating more frequently than usual and has told her mum it hurts when she voids. She has been hot to touch and her mother denies associated vomiting or diarrhoea symptoms. She opens her bowels every 2–3 days and occasionally strains. Her appetite has reduced today, although fluid intake is normal. She had an unremarkable birth history, and no known chronic medical issues, although she has had antibiotics on two occasions by her GP for urinary tract infections. She does not take any regular medications and immunisations are up to date.

Examination

The patient has a temperature of 37.7°C. Her cardiorespiratory observations are within normal limits. She is miserable but distractible during examination. She is well hydrated. She has a slightly distended but soft abdomen with no obvious focal tenderness or guarding. There is no organomegaly, but there is some possible faecal loading in the lower abdomen. She has normal external female genitalia. The rest of the examination is unremarkable.

 Investigations

- A clean catch urine sample is obtained and a dipstick test is performed: pH normal, nitrites +, leukocytes ++, ketones +, protein trace, blood negative and glucose negative.

Questions

1. What is the diagnosis?
2. What further investigations must be performed in the Emergency Department?
3. Outline the key principles in treating this patient.

DISCUSSION

This patient appears to have a lower urinary tract infection, which may be recurrent when taking the history into account.

The two broad clinical categories of urinary tract infections are pyelonephritis (upper urinary tract infection) and cystitis (lower urinary tract infections). The most common causative organisms are bowel flora, typically Gram-negative rods such as *E. coli.*

Children may be prone to urine infections due to factors such as constipation, bowel and bladder dysfunction, alteration of the periurethral flora by antibiotic therapy or, rarely, an anatomic anomaly such as posterior urethral valves. Female infants have a two- to- fourfold higher prevalence of UTI than male infants, thought to be due to a shorter urethra.

Clinical features can include fever, abdominal pain, nausea, vomiting, irritability, strong-smelling urine, enuresis, increased frequency of urination and dysuria. Infants may present only with failure to thrive.

This patient has symptoms suggestive of cystitis and has a positive dipstick result. A clean-catch sample should be sent for urgent microscopy and culture regardless of the dipstick result based on her age (less than 3 years old) and specific urinary symptoms alone. There are no indications based on the history or examination for other investigations in the Emergency Department.

The NICE guidance (UTI in under 16s) has further advice regarding interpretation of dipstick results and indications for culture. She should be commenced on oral antibiotics as first-line treatment. Common antibiotic choices include trimethoprim, nitrofurantoin, a cephalosporin or amoxicillin as advised by local departmental guidelines. This child may have had previous urine samples sent to the laboratory by her general practitioner. It would be advisable to seek these results and aim treatment based on previous sensitivities (if known). Toilet hygiene should be emphasised, e.g. girls should wipe from front to back, and wear loose cotton underwear.

In this case, it is also important to address the issue of her underlying constipation, with advice regarding diet and fluid intake, and consideration of the use of laxatives.

This patient is now considered to have recurrent UTIs based on three episodes of cystitis and warrants further outpatient investigation (ultrasound scan within 6 weeks and DMSA scan 4–6 months following the acute infection) to identify whether there is an underlying predisposition to infection and whether she has had subsequent renal tissue scarring.

If this patient can tolerate oral antibiotics and is clinically stable on assessment in the Emergency Department, discharge can be considered. Advice regarding when to return to the department should be provided, including if she becomes more unwell, has vomiting episodes and reduced fluid intake.

 Key Points

- Female infants have a higher prevalence of UTI than male infants.
- All patients less than 3 years of age should have a urine sample sent for urgent microscopy and culture regardless of the dipstick result.
- In addition to antibiotic treatment, ensure advice is provided regarding toilet hygiene and address possible underlying causes, such as constipation.

History

A 10-year-old presents with a 2-day history of worsening cough, and woke up this morning with shortness of breath. His mother tried to administer 10 puffs of salbutamol inhaler but with little effect, and so she called for an ambulance. He was born at term with an unremarkable birth history. He had eczema as an infant and currently uses salbutamol and beclometasone inhalers for his asthma. He has been requiring his salbutamol inhalers more regularly over the past couple of days. There is a strong family history of atopy. Immunisations are up to date.

Examination

His respiratory rate is 35–40 breaths/minute; he has oxygen saturation of 92% in air, heart rate of 110–130 beats/minute, systolic blood pressure of 90–110 mmHg, and he is afebrile. He is unable to perform a peak flow test.

The patient is breathless and finds it difficult to finish his sentences. On auscultation, there is bilateral end expiratory wheeze with reduced air entry at the bases. His cardiac and abdominal examinations are unremarkable.

Questions

1. What is the diagnosis?
2. What further investigations should be performed in the Emergency Department?
3. How would you manage this child?

DISCUSSION

This child is having a severe asthma attack and should be managed in the resuscitation area of the Emergency Department.

Asthma is one of the most common chronic diseases of childhood in the United Kingdom, and exacerbations are frequently encountered in the Emergency Department. Clinical features include cough, wheeze and breathlessness, which are secondary to bronchospasm, bronchial inflammation and mucosal oedema. Viral upper respiratory tract infections are the most common triggers for an acute exacerbation. Other predisposing factors include cold or humid weather, exercise and allergens. Asthma is strongly associated with other atopic conditions such as eczema and hayfever.

Differentials of wheeze include anaphylaxis, foreign body inhalation (causing a localised wheeze), congestive cardiac failure and gastro-oesophageal reflux and tracheal and bronchial anomalies in infants.

Diagnosis is usually based on clinical assessment and management initiated accordingly (Table 83.1).

A chest radiograph is not usually indicated unless there are concerns regarding pneumothorax, lobar collapse or consolidation and/or life-threatening asthma not responding to treatment.

Arterial blood gas measurements are not routinely required. They should be considered if there are life-threatening features not responding to treatment. Normal or raised pCO_2 levels are indicative of worsening asthma.

Children with severe or life-threatening asthma should receive frequent doses of nebulised salbutamol driven by oxygen. If there is a poor response, subsequent doses can be administered in combination with an anticholinergic, ipratropium bromide.

Steroids should be administered in the form of prednisolone (30–40 mg for children >5 years). Those already receiving maintenance steroid tablets could be given an extra dose of prednisolone. The dose of prednisolone should be repeated in those who vomit, or intravenous steroids like hydrocortisone should be considered. Treatment for up to 3 days is usually advised.

If there is poor response, treatment can be escalated in the form of intravenous salbutamol, intravenous magnesium sulphate and intravenous aminophylline. If the patient remains unstable despite this, intubation and ventilation will be required, and the patient will need to be transferred to an Intensive Care Unit.

Table 83.1 **Classification of asthma severity**

Moderate exacerbation	Severe exacerbation	Life threatening asthma
1. SpO$_2$ ≥ 92% 2. PEF ≥ 50% best or predicted 3. No clinical features of severe asthma	• SpO$_2$ < 92% • PEF < 50% best or predicted • Heart rate 120/min • Respiratory rate > 30/min • Use of accessory neck muscles • Too breathless to eat or complete sentences	• SpO$_2$ < 92% • Plus any of the following: • PEF < 33% best or predicted • Silent chest • Poor respiratory effort • Altered consciousness • Cyanosis • Exhaustion

If this patient responds to initial management and is felt to be appropriately stable, he can be transferred to the ward for inpatient care. The salbutamol dose should then be weaned to one- to two-hourly intervals, according to clinical response, and then weaned further towards four hourly intervals. The ipratropium bromide dose should be weaned to four- to six-hourly or discontinued.

Patients can be switched to inhaler and spacer treatment once improving on two- to four-hourly salbutamol.

 Key Points

- Acute asthma is a clinical diagnosis and does not require routine chest radiography or arterial blood gas analysis, unless there are signs of severe/life-threatening disease, or if an alternative chest pathology is possible (e.g. pneumothorax).
- Treatment includes the use of bronchodilators and anticholinergics such as salbutamol and ipratroprium bromide, respectively. Oral or intravenous steroids are also appropriate.
- In patients with severe exacerbations or not responding to initial therapy, consider intravenous malgesium sulphate or salbutamol.

CASE 84: A CHILD WITH DIFFICULTY FEEDING

History

An 8-week-old male infant presents with worsening vomiting after feeds. His parents have noticed that he arches his back and cries inconsolably after his feed. The vomits are non-projectile, with no blood or bile. He is having a mixture of breast feeds and formula feeds since birth, and takes these regularly. He is wetting his nappies as normal, and bowels open two to three times daily with soft stools. He is a first-born child. There were no significant antenatal or perinatal concerns. He has been otherwise well. He is due his first set of immunisations this week. There is no significant family history.

Examination

His cardiorespiratory observations in the Emergency Department were all within normal limits, and he is apyrexial. He handles well with an unremarkable examination. He is well hydrated and has a soft, non-tender abdomen with no obvious organomegaly.

Questions

1. What are the diagnosis and its underlying pathophysiology?
2. How would you manage this patient in the Emergency Department?

DISCUSSION

This patient has a clinical history suggestive of gastro-oesophageal reflux disease (GORD).

Reflux describes the passage of gastric contents into the oesophagus with or without regurgitation and vomiting. This is a very common, normal, physiological process and occurs in 5% of babies up to six times per day. GORD presents when reflux causes troublesome symptoms or complications. This has a prevalence of 10%–20%, and there is a higher risk in certain population groups such as premature babies and children with neurological impairments, oesophageal atresia and congenital diaphragmatic hernia.

Clinical features in infants include feed refusal, recurrent vomiting, poor weight gain, irritability and respiratory problems such as recurrent wheeze or cough. It rarely causes episodes of apnoea or acute life-threatening events. Ensure to exclude 'red-flag' symptoms such as haematemesis or bilious vomiting, which would suggest a different pathology.

Differentials for recurrent vomiting in this age group include cow's milk protein allergy, intestinal motility disorders, pyloric stenosis, infectious causes such as gastroenteritis and urinary tract infections and metabolic disorders.

No investigations are required in the Emergency Department if there is a suspicion of GORD; this is usually a clinical diagnosis alone. Outpatient investigations may include oesophageal pH study with impedance monitoring or upper GI contrast studies if there is suspected recurrent aspiration pneumonia, unexplained apnoeas, unexplained nonepileptic seizure-like events or persistent or faltering growth associated with overt regurgitation.

The parents should be advised to position the child in the upright position for 30 minutes after feeds. Contrary to advice given to adults with GORD, the child should sleep supine rather than the semi-supine position, as the latter is associated with Sudden Infant Death Syndrome.

In breastfeeding infants with feeding difficulties, ensure that the mother has had a breast-feeding assessment by a trained member of the staff. This will likely need to be arranged on an outpatient basis with the maternity department. If this continues despite a breastfeeding assessment and advice, consider alginate therapy (e.g. Gaviscon), for a trial period of 1–2 weeks, and continue if providing benefit.

In those who are formula-fed, firstly reduce the feed volume if it is thought to be excessive for the infant's weight. If appropriate, offer a trial of smaller, more frequent feeds (whilst ensuring an appropriate total daily amount of milk). If this regime is already in place, a trial of thickened formula (for example, containing rice starch, cornstarch, locust bean gum or carob bean gum) may provide benefit. If this is unsuccessful, stop the thickened formula and offer alginate therapy for a trial period of 1–2 weeks.

Consider a trial of a proton-pump inhibitor or histamine receptor antagonist if the above measures are unsuccessful. Beyond this, for severe and persisting symptoms, options include enteral tube feeding and fundoplication surgery.

Key Points

- GORD presents when reflux causes troublesome symptoms or complications. This has a prevalence of 10%–20%.
- GORD is a clinical diagnosis and does not require specific investigations. Clinical features include feed refusal, recurrent vomiting, poor weight gain, irritability and respiratory problems such as recurrent wheeze or cough.
- Initial management is conservative, including adequate feed volumes and positioning.
- Unlike adults with GORD, infants should still sleep in the supine position to mitigate the risk of Sudden Infant Death Syndrome.

History

A 3-year-old presents with a head injury that occurred when he fell off a chair onto a solid tiled floor approximately 2 hours ago. He cried immediately at which point his mother ran into the kitchen. There was no associated loss of consciousness. He was fully alert on her arrival and was given paracetamol as he was complaining of headache. He has 'been miserable' since and has had three discrete episodes of vomiting at home and one more in the Emergency Department. He has no significant medical history. There are no concerns relating to non-accidental injury.

Examination

His cardiorespiratory observations are all within normal limits and he is apyrexial. The child is quiet but alert and following commands. He is well hydrated. He has a small swelling, 4 cm in diameter, on the right temporal region, but no obvious signs of trauma elsewhere. His Glasgow Coma Scale is 14 (E4 V4 M6) 2 hours after the injury, and he has an otherwise normal neurological and fundoscopic examination.

Questions
1. What are the guidelines for a CT head scan?
2. What advice would you give a patient being discharged with a head injury?
3. How would you raise concerns about non-accidental injury?

DISCUSSION

This child has sustained a head injury and has now had three discrete episodes of vomiting following the incident. He does have a swelling in his temporal region and is quiet; however, the rest of his examination is unremarkable.

Head trauma is a very common presentation in children with falls being the most common cause. Most episodes are minor and not associated with brain injury or long-term sequelae.

Clinical features of concern in head injuries include multiple episodes of vomiting, which may reflect raised intracranial pressure. Other features include significant scalp haematoma, prolonged loss of consciousness, confusion and seizures.

Emergency Departments in the United Kingdom follow the NICE guidelines on indications for CT scanning in head injuries. A non-contrast CT scan of the brain is indicated in this child because he has four discrete episodes of vomiting and a GCS of 14, 2 hours after the injury. The scan should be performed within 1 hour of presentation.

If there is any radiological evidence of intracranial pathology, then neurosurgical advice should be sought as early as possible.

Even if the CT scan of the brain was 'normal', the clinical picture suggests that this child requires a period of observation to see if he has further episodes of vomiting or a deterioration in neurological status (current GCS 14), which would prompt consideration of repeat scanning.

Patients should only be discharged when they have returned to their baseline function and in the absence of significant ongoing headache. The parents should be fully informed of signs that warrant a return to the Emergency Department for another medical review. This includes further vomiting, change in behaviour, drowsiness, unconsciousness, problems in speaking/walking/with balance, weakness, seizures or clear fluid discharging from the ear or nose.

Any social concerns should be identified in the Emergency Department and discussion with social services undertaken if appropriate. Many children of this age presenting to the Emergency Department with trauma, but no other social concerns, may warrant a health visitor referral and information may be shared with the Child Protection team.

 Key Points

- Head injuries are common in children, but there are concerning features that warrant further investigation. These are outlined in the NICE guidelines on head injuries.
- If being discharged, patients should be given comprehensive advice on what symptoms warrant return to the Emergency Department. These are also outlined in the NICE guidelines, and most Emergency Departments have a head injury leaflet to give to patients.
- Non-accidental injury should be escalated via the paediatric or child protection team, depending on local policy.

History

A 2-year-old female presents with coryza and cough for the past 2 weeks, which is worsening in nature. She tends to have paroxysmal bouts of forceful coughing with vomiting. She has had three such episodes today, and these are worse at night. She has had mild pyrexia at home, and there is no associated difficulty in breathing. She has been more irritable, tired and anorexic for the last few days. There is no associated diarrhoea. She is passing urine as normal. She is generally fit and well, and does not take regular medications. The birth history was unremarkable. Her parents are separated; her father does not think she is up to date with her immunisations, as her mother declined some due to fear of complications.

Examination

Her temperature is 37.8°C. Her cardiorespiratory parameters are within normal limits. She has managed oral fluids in the department without further vomits.

The child is tearful on examination. She has dry mucous membranes, with a normal central capillary refill time. Her cardiovascular, respiratory and abdominal examinations are unremarkable. She has rhinitis, with enlarged, erythematous tonsils. Otoscopy is normal.

Questions

1. What are the diagnosis and its underlying pathophysiology?
2. What further assessment and investigations must be performed in the Emergency Department?
3. Outline the key principles in treating this patient.

DISCUSSION

The history of prolonged cough with paroxysms and vomiting, and the confusion surrounding the patient's immunisation status, should raise suspicion that this child may have pertussis, also known as whooping cough.

This is a very contagious respiratory illness caused by *Bordetella pertussis*. Patients are most contagious up to about 2 weeks after the cough begins, although antibiotics may shorten the period of time of infectivity.

In the twentieth century, pertussis was one of the most common childhood diseases and a major cause of childhood mortality. Since use of the immunisation began, incidence has decreased more than 75%. However, there has recently been an increase in the number of cases, which may be due to increased awareness and recognition of pertussis, greater access to laboratory diagnostic tools, increased reporting of pertussis to public health departments, and reduced immunity from vaccines, due to mutations of *Bordetella pertussis* at a genetic level.

The DTaP (Diptheria, Tetanus and Pertussis) vaccine is recommended for infants and children as per the UK immunisation schedule, and immunisation is now also advised for pregnant women during the 27th–36th week to provide transplacental antibody cover for newborns (the child still needs to have the immunisation when born).

The disease usually starts with coryza and a mild cough or pyrexia. After 1 to 2 weeks and as the disease progresses, symptoms may include coughing paroxysms followed by a high-pitched 'whoop', vomiting during or after coughing fits and tiredness or lethargy. The coughing fits can go on for up to 10 weeks or more, which is why it is also called the '100-day cough'.

Infants may present with apnoea, a known complication for those less than 6 months of age in particular, which is why pregnant women are encouraged to have the vaccine. Other complications of pertussis include otitis media, pneumonia, seizures and encephalopathy. There are also complications due to increased intra-thoracic and intra-abdominal pressure due to violent and/or prolonged coughing, such as pneumothorax, umbilical and inguinal hernias, rectal prolapse, subconjunctival or scleral haemorrhage and facial and truncal petechiae.

The diagnosis can be confirmed via nasopharyngeal aspirate/per nasal swabs, or detection of anti-pertussis toxin immunoglobulin G in blood or oral fluid samples. These should be taken in the Emergency Department before antibiotics are administered.

Admission will be required for patients who are 6 months of age or younger and acutely unwell, patients with significant breathing difficulties (e.g. apnoeic episodes, severe paroxysms or cyanosis) and patients with a significant complication (e.g. seizures or pneumonia). These patients will need respiratory isolation. Frequent vomiting can lead to dehydration; therefore, it is important to assess the child's hydration status and consider admission for IV fluids and antibiotics if warranted.

If the patient is discharged, which is usually the case, prescribe an antibiotic if the onset of cough is within the previous 21 days. A macrolide antibiotic such as azithromycin or clarithromycin is recommended first-line. Advise rest, adequate fluid intake and analgesia for symptomatic relief. Children who have suspected or confirmed whooping cough should stay off nursery or school for 5 days after starting antibiotics, or 21 days after the onset of cough (whichever is sooner).

Pertussis is a notifiable disease; the local Public Health England (PHE) centre should be informed of any suspicion of infection. Certain contact groups will also require prophylactic antibiotics in confirmed cases – please refer to the NICE guidelines/CDC website for further guidance.

 Key Points

- Pertussis is a notifiable disease. A vaccination exists for infants and pregnant mothers.
- It presents with a prolonged cough, with paroxysms, and vomiting. It is called the '100-day cough'.
- Its incubation period is around 3 weeks from the onset of the cough.
- Treatment includes macrolide antibiotics, which shorten the period of infectivity, and supportive management.

CASE 87: A CHILD WITH A PROLONGED FIT

History

A 10-year-old girl is brought into the Emergency Department resuscitation room following her first generalised tonic–clonic seizure. Her parents describe a 'strange noise' from her bedroom and found the patient in bed unconscious with jerking movements of the upper and lower limbs. This was associated with urinary incontinence. An ambulance was called immediately, and a dose of buccal midazolam was administered on their arrival, which terminated this episode. She had been well in herself during the day, and her parents do not think she had ingested alcohol, medications or illicit drugs prior to this episode. The child had no perinatal complications and is otherwise fit and well. Her maternal uncle was diagnosed with epilepsy as a child.

Examination

The patient is afebrile, with heart rate of 110–120 beats/minute, systolic blood pressure of 110–130 mmHg, respiratory rate of 25–30 breaths/minute and saturation of 100% on room air. The patient is asleep but responding to voice. Respiratory, cardiac and abdominal examinations are unremarkable. Her pupils are equal and reactive to light. She has normal tone and reflexes in her limbs. Blood glucose is 11 mmol/L.

Questions

1. What is the diagnosis and the underlying pathophysiology?
2. What further assessment and investigations must be performed in the Emergency Department?

DISCUSSION

The patient has had a prolonged afebrile seizure. She has not been known to have seizures in the past. Prolonged convulsive epileptic seizure should be diagnosed if a convulsive seizure with loss of consciousness/responsiveness has persisted for more than 5 minutes, or if there is no awakening between shorter repetitive seizures for the same period of time.

Prolonged seizures occur because of failure of the normal mechanisms that limit the spread and recurrence of seizure activity; this may be because excitation is excessive and/or inhibition is ineffective.

Causes of non-febrile seizures include epilepsy, metabolic or electrolyte disturbances, traumatic brain injury, intoxication and poisoning. An infectious cause should be considered if there is a recent history of pyrexia or being unwell.

The approach to the child who presents with a tonic–clonic convulsion lasting more than 5 minutes should be the same as the child who is in established status epilepticus. The primary aim should be to stop the seizure and to prevent the development of status epilepticus, which is defined as a seizure or cluster of seizures lasting 30 minutes.

The initial management of prolonged seizures is as per the Advanced Paediatric Life Support (APLS) protocol. The airway should be protected either by lying on the child on their side, insertion of an oropharngeal airway or, if the seizure is prolonged, involving an anaesthetist who may consider oro-tracheal intubation. The glucose level should be checked to exclude hypoglycaemia as a cause. Urea, electrolytes, calcium and magnesium should also be checked and blood cultures considered, depending on the history. Support blood pressure and correct electrolyte disturbances with fluids, if appropriate.

If the seizure is continuing beyond 5 minutes, the first-line medication is buccal midazolam or rectal diazepam at 0.5 mg/kg. If the patient has intravenous or intraosseous access, parenteral lorazepam can be administered as an alternative at 0.1 mg/kg – but IV access should not delay administration of anti-epileptic medication.

If the seizure continues after 10 minutes, repeat the above step of administering midazolam or diazepam. At this point, it is important to try and secure intravenous or intraosseous access. The patient should be closely monitored for signs of respiratory depression after giving benzodiazepines with end-tidal wave capnography useful in this regard.

If the seizure is not yet controlled 20 minutes after starting, the anaesthetic/intensive care teams should consider definitive airway control. An infusion of phenytoin should be commenced at 20 mg/kg over 20 minutes, or phenobarbitone if the patient already takes phenytoin. Phenytoin is an anti-epileptic that acts to slow down nerve conduction velocity and stabilises the cell membrane by inhibiting sodium influx. Phenobarbitone is a barbiturate that increases the effect of inhibitory GABA receptors.

Beyond this, if the seizure is refractory, rapid sequence induction (RSI) with thiopentone and intubation and ventilation will need to be considered. The patient will need to be admitted into a higher dependency unit or intensive care unit.

Consider a contrast enhanced CT head +/– lumbar puncture if seizures are atypical or focal, or if the aetiology is uncertain to rule out meningo-encephalits, brain abscess or space occupying lesion.

🔑	Key Points

- Seizures have many causes, many of which are reversible such as glucose and electrolyte disturbances.
- Seizures lasting more than 5 minutes, or cluster seizures that last less than 2 minutes but recur frequently, warrant the use of anticonvulsant medication such as buccal midazolam, rectal diazepam or intravenous lorazapam.
- In prolonged seizures, involve paediatric ICU and anaesthetist from an early stage to consider definitive airway management.

OBSTETRICS AND GYNAECOLOGY

CASE 88: VOMITING IN PREGNANCY

History

A 29-year-old primigravida woman presents to the Emergency Department with a 4-day history of persistent vomiting. She is 11 weeks pregnant with dichorionic diamniotic twins by spontaneous conception. She reports that she has been vomiting in excess of 15 times over the last 24 hours and is now unable to tolerate fluids as well as food. She has not opened her bowels over the last 2 days and is feeling very weak and lightheaded. She has had no vaginal bleeding but does have generalised low-grade upper abdominal pain with an occasional burning sensation in her chest. She is a non-smoker and has no significant past medical or surgical history.

Examination

She appears exhausted with dry mucus membranes. She is afebrile with a heart rate of 97 bpm and respiratory rate of 16. Her blood pressure drops from 100/79 mmHg (lying) to 90/65 on standing. The abdomen is soft, non-distended and mildly tender in the epigastrium. She has active bowel sounds.

 | Investigations

- *Urinalysis:* +4 ketones, nitrites negative, leucocytes negative, protein negative, glucose negative
- *Urinary pregnancy test:* Positive
- *Blood tests:* Hb 11.0, WCC 7.5, Na 135, K 2.9, Ur 7.1, Cr 60, ALT 29, ALP 270, GGT 30, Bilirubin 11, TSH 2, free T4 14

Questions

1. What is the most likely diagnosis and what are the possible differential diagnoses?
2. Name four risk factors associated with this condition.
3. Outline the key steps in managing this patient.

DISCUSSION

This patient is suffering with hyperemesis gravidarum, which accounts for one of the most common indications for hospital admission. It is defined as severe or long-lasting nausea and vomiting, appearing for the first time within the first trimester of pregnancy, and is so severe that weight loss, dehydration and electrolyte imbalance may occur. It affects less than 4% of pregnant women, although up to 80% of women suffer from some degree of nausea and vomiting throughout their pregnancy. Although the pathophysiology is poorly understood, it is thought to be associated with rising levels of human chorionic gonadotrophin (hCG) hormone. Therefore, conditions that give rise to exaggerated levels of hCG such as multiple pregnancy and trophoblastic disease are risk factors. Other risk factors include obesity, nulliparous women and a previous history of hyperemesis gravidarum or motion sickness.

Classically, patients present with a long history of nausea and vomiting that becomes progressively worse, despite treatment with simple antiemetics. They are unable to keep down any food or fluids and attend looking severely dehydrated. They may have lost over 5% of their pre-pregnancy weight and will have evidence of ketonuria.

Other medical or surgical causes of nausea and vomiting must be excluded when making a diagnosis of hyperemesis gravidarum. Conditions such as peptic ulcer disease, bowel obstruction, pancreatitis, gastroenteritis, cholecystitis, appendicitis, hepatitis and a urinary tract infection are differentials that must be considered. Metabolic conditions such as thyrotoxicosis and drug-induced nausea and vomiting are also other conditions that should be kept in mind.

Investigations are required to rule out other causes of nausea and vomiting. The Pregnancy-Unique Quantification of Emesis (PUQE) can be used as an objective measure to classify the severity of nausea and vomiting. Basic blood tests include full blood count, electrolytes (including calcium and phosphate) and liver and thyroid function tests. A venous blood gas can be performed in diabetics to exclude diabetic ketoacidosis. Urinalysis can be used to investigate the degree of urinary ketones and the presence or absence of an infection. An ultrasound scan should be scheduled in the gynaecology department to confirm viability and gestational age, as well as to exclude a multiple pregnancy or trophoblastic disease. Severe abdominal pain may warrant further investigation with a serum amylase, an abdominal ultrasound or an oesophageal gastroduodenoscopy, if deemed appropriate.

The treatment of hyperemesis gravidarum is mainly supportive, as it is a self-limiting condition. However, treatment is required to avoid future complications such as hyponatraemia, hypokalaemia and Wernicke's encephalopathy and to allow the patient to get back to her activities of daily living. Management involves rehydration with intravenous fluids supplemented with potassium to correct the hypokalaemia, initially given quickly over 2–4 hours. Dextrose is contraindicated in these patients as it may precipitate encephalopathy and worsen hyponatraemia. Antiemetics should be given intravenously or intramuscularly if unable to be taken orally. Cyclizine is considered first-line anti-emetic and metoclopramide is used as second-line treatment. Ondansetron is often considered as third-line. Gastric protection with ranitidine and vitamin supplementation using IV thiamine (pabrinex) initially, followed by oral thiamine and folic acid, is given to prevent possible complications. Whilst inpatient, thromboprophylaxis is required in the form of low-molecular-weight heparin and compression stockings as these women are at high risk of a venous thromboembolism secondary to pregnancy, immobility and dehydration. Rarely, nutritional supplementation (enteral or parenteral) and corticosteroids are required in intractable severe cases of hyperemesis.

Ambulatory daycare management is suitable for most patients who are unable to tolerate oral antiemetics or fluids. Inpatient management should be considered in those with a severe electrolyte abnormality, significant co-morbidities or recurrent episodes of nausea and vomiting or hyperemesis gravidarum. Women who have vomiting but who are not dehydrated or can tolerate medications orally can be managed within the community.

🔑	Key Points
	• Hyperemesis gravidarum is more common with family history, trophoblastic disease and multiple pregnancy.
	• Assess all women for dehydration and electrolyte disturbance.
	• Give anti-emetics, intravenous fluid and vitamins to those unable to tolerate oral intake.
	• Perform an ultrasound scan to rule out trophoblastic disease if before the 12 week routine dating scan.
	• Remember to give VTE thromboprophylaxis to those that are admitted into hospital.

History

A 26-year-old woman comes in to the Emergency Department complaining of severe sharp lower abdominal pain, worse on the right-hand side. She has vomited twice and is feeling dizzy with some right shoulder tip pain. She is gravida 0 para 0 and thinks that her last menstrual period was around 7 weeks ago. She reports having a small amount of brown vaginal spotting this morning. She is sexually active and has the copper intrauterine contraceptive device (IUCD) in situ. Five years ago, she was treated for chlamydia but has no other past medical history. Her last cervical smear was 1 year ago and was normal. She has never had any surgery and does not smoke.

Examination

She appears pale and is evidently in pain despite having been given analgesia. Vital signs show a temperature of 37.5°C, heart rate of 115, respiratory rate of 20, blood pressure of 91/63 mmHg and oxygen saturation of 97% on room air. Her abdomen is not distended, but she is generally tender, especially in the right iliac fossa where she has voluntary guarding. On speculum and bimanual examination, the cervix appears normal and closed. There is no fresh blood or discharge seen. She has a normal-sized anteverted uterus; however, it is found to have cervical tenderness and is extremely tender in the right adenexa.

Investigations
• *Urinalysis:* Ketones negative, nitrites negative, leucocytes negative, protein negative, glucose negative.
• *Blood tests:* Hb 9.8, MCV 91, WCC 9.2, Plts 407.

Questions

1. What is the first investigation that you would like to perform in this patient and what other investigations are required?
2. What is your working diagnosis and differential diagnoses?
3. How should this patient be managed within the Emergency Department?

DISCUSSION

In a female of reproductive age, this is an ectopic pregnancy until proven otherwise. As there is evidence of haemodynamic compromise, it is likely that this has ruptured and should be managed as a gynaecological emergency in the resuscitation room.

An ectopic pregnancy is any pregnancy that has implanted outside of the endometrial cavity and occurs in around 1% of pregnancies with an estimated 11,000 ectopic pregnancies diagnosed each year within the United Kingdom. By far the most common site of implantation for an ectopic pregnancy is within the fallopian tube, accounting for around 95% of ectopics. Less commonly, a pregnancy can implant within the ovary (0.5%), the cervix (<1%), a caesarean section scar (<1%) or the abdominal cavity (1%). Risk factors include a previous ectopic pregnancy, a history of pelvic inflammatory disease or infertility, in vitro fertilisation, the presence of an IUCD, previous tubal damage or surgery and smoking.

Women may present with acute onset unilateral abdominal/pelvic pain, associated with nausea and vomiting and a history of amenorrhoea with a positive pregnancy test. They may or may not have had some vaginal spotting. Signs and symptoms of dizziness, shoulder-tip pain, tachycardia, hypotension and peritonism suggest a haemoperitoneum and therefore a ruptured ectopic. Classic features that may be elicited on bimanual examination include cervical excitation and marked adnexal tenderness. If a woman is stable and has an intact ectopic pregnancy, she may just present with a mild to moderate amount of pain with some possible vaginal bleeding.

You must consider all causes of an acute abdomen. The differential diagnosis includes appendicitis, ovarian torsion, ruptured ovarian cyst, renal colic, endometriosis and pelvic inflammatory disease.

A pregnancy test is the first investigation required in all women of reproductive age to determine whether the abdominal pain may be pregnancy or non-pregnancy related. Other essential baseline investigations include baseline blood tests (full blood count, electrolytes, serum β-hCG), urinalysis and a venous blood gas to measure levels of acidosis and lactate and for a quick measure of the patient's haemoglobin. A serum progesterone is not useful in predicting an ectopic pregnancy. Transvaginal ultrasound is the diagnostic investigation of choice in the case of a stable ectopic pregnancy, which has a reported sensitivity of 87%–99% and specificity of 94%–99%. In an unstable patient where rupture is suspected, patients should be taken straight to the operating theatre for a diagnostic laparoscopy.

This patient must be taken straight through for immediate resuscitation; laid flat with high flow oxygen through a non-rebreathe facial mask. She requires IV access with two large-bore cannulae and intravenous fluid given immediately. She will need 4 units of blood cross-matched, and if severely haemodynamically compromised, O negative blood can be given immediately to avoid delay. This patient requires consent for a diagnostic laparoscopy or laparotomy and salpingectomy and a quick transfer to theatre. Anti-D prophylaxis should be offered to all Rhesus-negative women who have a surgical removal of an ectopic or with repeated vaginal bleeding.

Point-of-care ultrasonography is useful in the Emergency Department (FAST protocol) and can be used to look for intra-abdominal free fluid and in same cases can be used to confirm the presence or absence of an intrauterine pregnancy, depending on gestation. Caution must be exercised to use this as a rule-in strategy as small volumes (<150 mL) of free fluid may not be visualised.

This patient is clearly unwell and requires admission and surgery as a matter of urgency. In cases where the patient is stable and an intact ectopic is suspected, this is not an emergency and patients can be brought back the next day for an ultrasound scan in the gynaecology department if seen out of hours. Dependent on scan findings and serum β-hCG levels, it is usually a consultant decision to advise on further treatment. This can be managed expectantly with serial β-hCG monitoring, medically with methotrexate or surgically with either a salpingotomy or salpingectomy.

🔑 | **Key Points**

- Abdominal pain and collapse with a positive pregnancy test must be treated as a ruptured ectopic pregnancy until proven otherwise.
- Manage shocked patients in the resuscitation room with fluids or packed red cells, analgesia and prompt referral to the gynaecology team.
- Point-of-care ultrasound is useful to rule in the presence of free fluid in the abdomen and rule-out an ectopic pregnancy in the presence of an intrauterine pregnancy.
- Definitive management can be medical or surgical and depends on the location of the ectopic pregnancy, age and haemodynamic status.

History

A 35-year-old gravida 1 para 0, woman presents to you in the Emergency Department with dark red vaginal bleeding over the last 7 hours. This initially started as light spotting, but over the last few hours, this has become heavier. She has passed some large clots and is having some cramping and lower abdominal pain. She took a home pregnancy test 9 weeks ago that was positive. She has a history of one previous miscarriage, requiring surgical management for retained products of conception. She has had a large-loop excision of the transformation zone (LLETZ) 3 years ago for an abnormal smear but has no other significant past medical or surgical history to note.

Examination

On examination, she is warm and well perfused with a heart rate of 84 bpm and blood pressure of 124/64 mmHg. Her abdomen is soft and non-tender. Speculum examination shows a closed cervix, which is normal in appearance, with some fresh blood coming through the vaginal canal. On bimanual examination, she has an anteverted 10-week sized uterus and no cervical excitation or adenexal tenderness. She is very anxious about her baby.

 Investigations

- *Urinary pregnancy test*: Positive.
- *Blood tests*: Hb 12.0, WCC 8.0, Rhesus negative.

Questions

1. What are the possible causes of bleeding in early pregnancy?
2. What is the most likely diagnosis and how would this be confirmed?
3. How would you manage this patient?

DISCUSSION

There should be a high index of suspicion of threatened miscarriage in this patient. A diagnosis of miscarriage can be made on the basis of a detailed history and examination or on ultrasound. Some women can have bleeding with a viable pregnancy. A miscarriage is a spontaneous loss of a pregnancy before viability at 24 weeks' gestation and is classified by clinical type (Table 90.1). It is common and occurs in 20% of clinical pregnancies with the majority of these occurring within the first trimester. Recurrent miscarriage affects 1% of women trying to conceive and is defined as the loss of three or more consecutive pregnancies. Risk factors for miscarriage include advanced maternal age, smoking, obesity, previous history of miscarriage and treatment to the cervix. Antiphospholipid syndrome is the most important treatable cause for recurrent miscarriage.

Women often present with a history of vaginal bleeding and cramp-like lower abdominal pain. They may only have very light bleeding, or they may report heavy bleeding, filling multiple pads and passing large clots. It is important to perform a speculum examination on these patients to assess whether the cervical os is open or closed and to look for other causes of vaginal bleeding. Some women may present with signs of shock or collapse following vaginal bleeding secondary to cervical shock. It is essential to examine these women with a speculum and remove any products of conception that may be stuck within the cervical canal causing reflex bradycardia and a vasovagal effect.

It is important to keep in mind all causes of vaginal bleeding and pelvic pain including cervical ectropion, cervical polyp, ectopic pregnancy, molar pregnancy, cervical carcinoma, urinary tract infection, appendicitis and a ruptured ovarian cyst.

Baseline investigations required within the Emergency Department include a urinary pregnancy test, a full blood count and group and screen to assess for anaemia and the patient's rhesus status. A venous blood gas may be performed if the patient is haemodynamically compromised or unwell and will give an indication of haemoglobin and lactate. Ultimately the patient will require a transvaginal ultrasound scan, which should be arranged with the gynaecology department as there are strict ultrasound criteria for diagnosing a miscarriage.

Table 90.1 **Classification of miscarriage**

Missed miscarriage	Ultrasound features of a non-viable or non-continuing pregnancy, despite the absence of clinical features.
Threatened miscarriage	Threat of miscarriage with unprovoked vaginal bleeding with or without abdominal pain. The cervical os is closed.
Incomplete miscarriage	Products of conception are only partially expelled and the cervical os is open.
Complete miscarriage	Products of conception are completely expelled. The cervical os is closed and the uterus is empty.
Inevitable miscarriage	Unprovoked vaginal bleeding and the cervical os is open.
Septic miscarriage	Products of conception from a missed or incomplete miscarriage become infected.
Recurrent miscarriage	Spontaneous loss of three or more consecutive pregnancies.

It is important to counsel these women on all options for management of miscarriage, including the risks and benefits of each. Options (depending on urgency and gestational size) include

1. *Expectant management, using a watch and wait approach.* This avoids medical intervention and can be managed at home. However, it is unpredictable and has a higher chance of retained products. It is usually more successful for incomplete miscarriages.
2. *Medical management, using vaginal (or oral) misoprostol.* This avoids surgical risks and can also be managed at home. However, it still holds risks of infection and heavy bleeding, and if it fails, patients may still require surgical intervention.
3. *Surgical management to evacuate retained products of conception (ERPC).* This is the least likely to fail and can be arranged in advance. Modern management now allows this to be performed under general anaesthetic or under local anaesthetic using manual vacuum aspiration (MVA). Nevertheless, these still hold the risks of surgical complications.

Women who are bleeding heavily or who are at increased risk of haemorrhage will require immediate surgical management to arrest the bleeding. Offer anti-D immunoglobulin to all women who are Rhesus negative and have surgical management of miscarriage and to women who are beyond 12 + 0 weeks of gestation. This precludes haemolytic disease of the fetus and newborn in future pregnancies.

Depending on trust policy, in-hours stable patients can usually be sent straight to the Early Pregnancy Assessment Unit (EPAU) for a scan. Out of hours you should liaise with the on-call gynaecology doctor. If the patient only has moderate bleeding and is otherwise well, she can normally be brought back the following day for a scan in the department.

She will be very distressed and it is important to keep her calm and not to diagnose a miscarriage without confirmation by ultrasound unless fetal points are seen. Once a diagnosis has been made, it is vital to express sympathy and provide adequate counselling. She must be reassured that miscarriages are common, that they are usually due to sporadic chromosomal abnormalities and that it is not a result of anything that she has done. It is important for her to know that although she has had two consecutive miscarriages, there is a very good chance that she will have a normal pregnancy in the future. Contact information and information leaflets can be given for support and counselling groups. All women who have recurrent miscarriages should be referred to the Recurrent Miscarriage Clinic for further investigation.

Advise that a repeat scan may be required after treatment if bleeding persists, if there are signs of infection or if bleeding does not start up to 2 weeks after expectant management.

 Key Points

- Bleeding in early pregnancy is common and does not necessarily lead to miscarriage.
- Assess all women with bleeding in early pregnancy along standard ED guidelines and resuscitate those that display signs of shock or large bleeds.
- Perform baseline blood investigations if bleeding is heavy.
- Stable patients with low-volume blood loss may be brought back to EPAU the next day.
- Patients with heavy bleeding or signs of shock should be managed in the resuscitation room and referred to the gynaecology team.
- Women and their partners will be emotionally distressed and should be treated with empathy and kindness.

CASE 91: PELVIC PAIN

History

A 16-year-old girl is brought in to the Emergency Department via ambulance. She reports a sudden onset left lower quadrant abdominal pain. Initially it was colicky in nature but now is constant and has greatly increased in severity. She feels hot and has vomited on four occasions. She has not had any urinary symptoms or change in bowel habit. She has not had any vaginal bleeding and is not currently sexually active. She has regular menstrual cycles and her last menstrual period was 1 week ago.

Examination

She appears flushed, unwell and in a lot of pain. She has a low-grade pyrexia at 37.7°C and is tachycardic at 113 bpm. Her blood pressure is 115/75 mmHg. She has generalised tenderness on abdominal palpation, but is worst in the left iliac fossa with associated rebound tenderness and guarding. On speculum examination, the vaginal canal and cervix are normal. Bimanual examination reveals severe pain in the left adnexa.

Investigations
• *Urinalysis:* Ketones negative, nitrites negative, leucocytes negative, protein negative, glucose negative.
• *Urinary pregnancy test:* Negative.
• *Blood tests:* Hb 12.0, WCC 8.0, Plts 398, CRP 45.

Questions

1. What is the most likely diagnosis that must be excluded?
2. How would you manage this patient?

DISCUSSION

This patient gives a classic presentation of ovarian cyst torsion. This involves the twisting of the ovary and the cyst on its pedicle, thereby blocking the vascular supply to the ovary eventually leading to ischaemia and necrosis of ovarian tissue. Anatomic changes in the weight and size of the ovary may alter the position of the fallopian tubes, making torsion more likely to occur. Torsion of the ovary and/or fallopian tube account for between 2.4% and 7.4% of all gynaecological emergencies, and rapid intervention is required in order to preserve ovarian function. It most commonly occurs in women of reproductive age, but can occur at any age.

Diagnosis can be difficult and is mainly based on clinical presentation. Acute onset of unilateral pelvic pain associated with nausea and vomiting are common presenting features. Pain may initially fluctuate secondary to intermittent torsion followed by severe constant pain from persistent torsion. Going further back into the history, they may have had intermittent episodes of pain for some time. On examination, these patients often have low-grade pyrexia, tachycardia, generalised abdominal tenderness and localised features of rebound and guarding. On vaginal examination, they may have signs of cervical excitation and adnexal tenderness or an adnexal mass may be palpable. However, in reality, a vaginal examination is often extremely difficult to perform as the woman is so tender.

It is important to take a detailed history in any women where ovarian torsion is suspected. Differential diagnoses include a ruptured ovarian cyst, ectopic pregnancy, pelvic inflammatory disease, appendicitis, renal colic and ovarian hyperstimulation syndrome.

Baseline investigations are required in any female presenting with an acute abdomen. It is essential to exclude an ectopic pregnancy with a urinary pregnancy test, and urinalysis should be performed to look for infection. Blood tests that must be taken are a full blood count, electrolytes, liver function and a group and save. Ovarian torsion is unfortunately often misdiagnosed due to its non-specific symptoms and lack of diagnostic tools. Transvaginal ultrasound using colour Doppler is first-line investigation and may indicate the presence of an ovarian cyst, in addition to an enlarged and oedematous ovary with absence of blood flow. Definitive diagnosis is surgical where there is a high index of suspicion. CT and MRI have been shown to be useful, especially the use of MRI in the second and third trimesters of pregnancy for diagnosing abdominal pain, when the ovaries and appendix are more difficult to visualise with ultrasound. However, in practice, this is almost never needed, as the presentation is usually clear and a transvaginal ultrasound scan usually confirms the diagnosis.

Initial resuscitation and stabilisation are required in all patients with an acute abdomen. Prompt intervention is required to preserve ovarian function. Recent evidence has concluded that laparoscopic surgery with de-torsion is the preferred treatment method in prepubescent girls and women of reproductive age to preserve normal ovarian function and fertility, regardless of the appearance of the ovary at the time of surgery. In older or postmenopausal women, oophorectomy is the treatment of choice to avoid future risk of re-torsion. If there is evidence of a non-functional cyst, a cystectomy should be performed at the time of surgery.

This is a gynaecological emergency and requires immediate attention, transfer to theatre and overnight admission. Patients with a suspected diagnosis of ovarian torsion should be admitted for gynaecological assessment, observation or surgical management.

Key Points

- Suspect ovarian torsion in women with severe sudden onset unilateral pelvic pain.
- Urinalysis is key to exclude a ruptured ectopic pregnancy.
- Transvaginal ultrasound is the imaging modality of choice to confirm the diagnosis.
- Definitive management is surgical with laparoscopic de-torsion or oophorectomy.

History

A 45-year-old woman attends the Emergency Department feeling feverish, nauseous and generally unwell over the last 3 days. She has been passing foul-smelling green vaginal discharge over the last 2 weeks and has recently developed increasing lower abdominal pain. She complains of deep dyspareunia, which has only started over the last week. She has been with her new partner for the last 4 months. Around 3 weeks ago, she was fitted with a copper IUCD. She does not have any urinary or bowel symptoms. She has had three normal vaginal deliveries in the past and no other pregnancies. Her cervical smears are up-to-date and normal. She has no history of sexually transmitted infections (STIs) in the past or any other significant medical or surgical history.

Examination

Vital signs: heart rate of 103 bpm, blood pressure of 100/65 mmHg, respiratory rate of 18 and temperature of 38.1°C. Her abdomen is soft but generally tender all across the lower abdomen. There is no guarding, rebound tenderness or rigidity. On speculum examination, there is malodorous green discharge seen originating from the cervix. On bimanual examination, cervical excitation is elicited and she has bilateral adnexal tenderness, more prominent on the left.

Questions

1. How would you investigate this lady?
2. What is the most likely diagnosis and cause of her symptoms?
3. Outline the key principles in treating this patient.

DISCUSSION

The most likely diagnosis in this patient is pelvic inflammatory disease (PID). PID is the clinical syndrome associated with an upper genital tract resulting from ascending infection from the endocervix. This can further lead to endometritis, salpingitis, parametritis, oophoritis, tuboovarian abscess and pelvic peritonitis. It is almost always a result of untreated STIs with *Chlamydia trachomatis* and *Neisseria gonorrhoea* being the leading causes of PID. Occasionally it can occur after a surgical procedure where the uterus is instrumented or following fitting of an intrauterine device. In 2011, Public Health England published data stating that the rate of diagnosed PID amongst 15–44 year olds within hospital settings was 241 per 100,000 compared to 176 per 100,000 in GP settings. Long-term complications can arise in women with PID including repeated pelvic infections, Fitz–Hugh–Curtis syndrome, tuboovarian abscess, ectopic pregnancy, infertility and long-term pelvic pain.

PID may be symptomatic or asymptomatic. Typical features that may be elicited from the history that are suggestive of PID include bilateral lower abdominal pain, deep dyspareunia, abnormal vaginal discharge and fever. Some women also report right upper quadrant pain and abnormal vaginal bleeding including post-coital and intermenstrual bleeding. On physical examination, the patient may be pyrexial and is usually tender across her lower abdomen. On bimanual examination, adnexal tenderness and cervical motion tenderness are common features.

Differential diagnosis of lower abdominal pain in young women includes ectopic pregnancy, endometriosis, appendicitis, ovarian cyst torsion or rupture and urinary tract infection.

A diagnosis of PID is mainly made on clinical grounds; however, it is firstly essential to rule out an ectopic pregnancy using a urinary pregnancy test. Urinalysis and blood tests including a full blood count, electrolytes and liver function should be performed in anyone with abdominal pain and suspected infection. In patients who are pyrexial, blood cultures and an arterial blood gas should also be performed. Endocervical swabs should be taken to look for gonorrhoea and chlamydia, as well as a high vaginal swab to investigate for other genital infections such as bacterial vaginosis and candidiasis. A transvaginal ultrasound scan of the pelvis may also be performed to investigate for other causes of pelvic pain and the presence of a tuboovarian abscess.

This woman needs to be admitted for broad-spectrum intravenous antibiotics according to trust policy and requires fluid resuscitation. Adequate analgesia should also be given. Evidence-based recommended inpatient regimes include IV ceftriaxone and IV/oral metronidazole along with oral doxycycline (or IV if not tolerated orally) and oral metronidazole. Alternatively, IV clindamycin and gentamicin initially, followed by either oral clindamycin or doxycycline plus oral metronidazole, may be given to complete a 14-day course. Intravenous therapy should be continued for 24 hours after clinical improvement and then stepped down to oral medication. In situations where improvement does not occur within 24–48 hours and a tuboovarian abscess is suspected, the patient may require a laparoscopy or laparotomy to confirm this and drain the abscess.

If a woman presents with PID and has either a copper or Mirena coil in situ, it should be discussed with the patient as to whether this should be removed. Removal should be considered if the patient requests it or if her symptoms have not resolved within 72 hours. If it is removed, you must find out from the patient whether she has had sexual intercourse in the last 7 days and whether she would like emergency contraception.

Clearly this patient is septic and therefore requires admission. Women with mild or moderate PID can be managed in the community with oral antibiotics. Delaying treatment of PID increases the risk of long-term complications and therefore a low threshold for empirical treatment of PID is recommended. Patients should be advised not to have unprotected intercourse until they and their partner(s) have completed the course of treatment and attended follow-up. The need for contact tracing, screening and treatment should be discussed to prevent reinfection. Women should be warned about the future risks of infertility, ectopic pregnancy and chronic pelvic pain, and that the future use of barrier contraception will significantly reduce the risk of PID.

Key Points
• PID may be caused by untreated sexually treated infections, instrumentation of the uterus or coil devices.
• Urinary pregnancy testing is important to rule out ectopic pregnancy.
• Transvaginal ultrasound may be required to look for a tubo-ovarian abscess or to exclude other ovarian pathology.
• Treatment is by 14 days of broad spectrum antibiotics according to local guidelines.

History

A 21-year-old woman comes in complaining of vulval pain and swelling. She says that she noticed a pea-sized swelling on her right vulva that appeared around 3 weeks ago, but she had not paid much attention. Over the last 2 days, it has rapidly increased in size and is now very large and painful. She is unable to walk or sit without feeling discomfort. She does not have any vaginal bleeding or discharge and has never had this before. She is sexually active and is using the combined oral contraceptive pill. She has no history of STIs or abnormal cervical smears and has never been pregnant.

Examination

On examination, her abdomen is soft and non-tender. She has a right labial swelling, which is extremely tender to touch and extends anteriorly from the level of the posterior introitus. It measures 7 × 5 × 4 cm and is erythematous, fluctuant and tense. She has a temperature of 37.5°C, a heart rate of 70 bpm, blood pressure of 123/78 mmHg and respiratory rate of 13 bpm.

Questions

1. What is the diagnosis?
2. How would you manage this patient?

DISCUSSION

This patient has a Bartholin's gland abscess. The greater vestibular glands, also known as Bartholin's glands, are situated at the base of the vestibular bulbs. They open out onto either side of the lower vagina at 5 and 7 o'clock positions and are important to provide lubrication during sexual intercourse. If a blockage occurs in either of the ducts, a tense cyst forms that commonly becomes infected due to their location forming an abscess. Bartholin's abscesses are polymicrobial and often contain *E. coli*, *Bacteriodes*, *Peptostreptococci* and *N. gonorrhoea*. Bartholin's duct cysts are relatively common, mainly affecting women within their reproductive years, and are seen in 2% of women presenting to gynaecological services.

Clinical features include a unilateral swelling near the posterior aspect of the vulva. This will be very painful especially on movement or sitting and will be erythematous and tense. It is important to establish if it is fluctuant and therefore whether it can be drained. The patient may also have a low-grade fever.

Other causes of vulval swellings include Bartholin's gland malignancy, vulval haematoma, mucous cyst of the vestibule, vulval fibroma, lipoma, sebaceous cyst and perianal abscess.

This is a clinical diagnosis and should be made based on history and examination. If the swelling is discharging fluid, a swab should be taken and sent to the laboratory for microscopy, culture and sensitivity. If the patient is pyrexial, blood tests including a full blood count, C-reactive protein and blood cultures may also be taken.

The abscess must be drained surgically and the pus sent for culture, as well as giving analgesia and a course of oral antibiotics. The most common method of drainage in the United Kingdom is via marsupialisation of the cyst/abscess. This involves making an incision and clearing the loculations within the cyst. Part of the cyst wall is then excised, and the edges are sutured to the skin to allow continued drainage, and subsequent healing from the base. The cavity may then be packed with ribbon gauze, which is removed within a few hours. Patients are usually followed up 6 weeks post-operatively. Alternatively, a Word catheter can be inserted into the abscess for 3–4 weeks, allowing continual drainage and epithelialisation of the tract thereby forming a long-term outflow route for the gland.

It is important to note that the area is highly vascular and there can be significant blood loss. Therefore, surgical intervention is usually reserved for a recurrent, large or multilocular cyst/abscess. Small asymptomatic cysts (measuring less than 2 cm) do not require surgical drainage and can be treated conservatively with warm baths, compressors, analgesia and a course of antibiotics.

If the patient is systemically well, she does not need admission. Depending on the severity of the patient's symptoms, it is possible to send patients away with a course of antibiotics and arrange for her to be brought back for an elective surgical procedure. Word catheters are inserted in the clinic and can be performed under local anaesthetic. It is important to inform patients that Bartholin's cysts/abscesses can reoccur and may require repeat treatment.

	Key Points
	• Bartholin's gland abscesses are caused by infected mucocoeles of the gland.
	• Small abscesses in well patients may be treated by warm baths and oral antibiotics.
	• Surgical treatment options include incision and drainage, marsupialisation or Word catheter insertion.
	• Patients should be warned of recurrence.

History

A 33-year-old lady presents to the Emergency Department with a distended abdomen and feeling breathless. She is gravida 1 para 0 and tells you that she is now 3 days' post egg retrieval for in vitro fertilisation (IVF). She initially noticed abdominal bloating; however, this has significantly increased over the last 2 days. She has been vomiting this morning and has found herself increasingly short of breath today. She has also noticed that she has been passing small amounts of dark urine over the last couple of days.

Examination

Vital signs: heart rate of 95 bpm, blood pressure of 105/70 mmHg, respiratory rate of 18, temperature of 36.9°C, O_2 saturation of 96% on room air. Respiratory examination reveals decreased air entry at the left base but heart sounds are normal. Her abdomen is distended and generally tender. Signs of both a fluid thrill and shifting dullness are elicited. She has bilateral ankle oedema.

Investigations
• *Blood tests:* Hb 11.0, WCC 8.0, Hct 0.5, Na 130, K 5.2, Ur 14, Cr 75, ALT 30, ALP 55, GGT 27, Bilirubin 10, albumin 24.
• *Chest x-ray:* Mild pleural effusion at left base. No collapse, consolidation or cardiomegaly.
• *Abdominal and pelvic ultrasound scan:* Bilaterally enlarged multicystic ovaries measuring 14 × 12 cm on the right and 15 × 13 cm on the left. There is a large volume of ascites. Otherwise no other abnormalities have been noted.

Questions

1. What is the diagnosis?
2. What complications may arise in these patients?
3. How should she be managed?

DISCUSSION

This patient has ovarian hyperstimulation syndrome (OHSS). OHSS is an iatrogenic complication of fertility treatment with exogenous gonadotrophins to promote oocyte formation. Hyperstimulation of the ovaries leads to ovarian enlargement, and subsequent exposure to human chorionic gonadotrophin (hCG) causes production of proinflammatory mediators, primarily vascular endothelial growth factor (VEGF). The effects of proinflammatory mediators lead to increased vascular permeability and a loss of fluid from intravascular to third space compartments. This gives rise to ascites, pleural effusions and in some cases pericardial effusions. Women with severe OHSS can typically lose up to 20% of their circulating volume in the acute phase leading to a reduced serum osmolality and sodium concentration, hence altering the threshold of antidiuretic hormone (ADH) release. OHSS patients are also at high risk of developing a thromboembolism as a result of haemoconcentration and immobilisation.

The incidence of OHSS varies depending on the type of fertility treatment. In conventional IVF, around one-third of cycles are affected by mild OHSS. The combined incidence of moderate or severe OHSS is reported as between 3.1% and 8%. Risk factors include a previous history of OHSS, age under 30 years, polycystic ovaries, increased antral follicle count and high levels of anti-Müllerian hormone (AMH).

Initially, patients with OHSS present with abdominal bloating secondary to ovarian enlargement, later followed by accumulation of abdominal ascites. This occurs following the injection used to promote final follicular maturation before oocyte retrieval. There may be a palpable mass per abdomen or signs and symptoms of intraperitoneal fluid. Nausea and vomiting are often associated with this. The decrease in intravascular volume gives rise to dehydration and haemoconcentration and leads to oliguria and thromboembolism in severe cases.

Once OHSS is suspected, the severity should be graded as mild, moderate, severe or critical according to the standardised classification scheme (Table 94.1).

Alternative differential diagnoses of abdominal pain and distension include intra-abdominal haemorrhage, pelvic inflammatory disease, ectopic pregnancy, appendicitis, haemorrhagic ovarian cyst, bowel perforation, liver disease, ovarian cyst torsion and rupture.

Patients should have a full workup including a full blood count, electrolytes, clotting profile, serum osmolality and C-reactive protein. The haematocrit and white cell count are of particular importance when grading severity. Urinalysis and a urinary pregnancy test should also be performed on all women of reproductive years that present with abdominal pain. Physical examination should include body weight and abdominal girth at the umbilicus. The patient should be assessed for the presence of ascites, pleural effusion and thrombosis in the form of a pulmonary embolism or deep vein thrombosis. Caution should be taken with pelvic examinations to avoid trauma to enlarged ovaries. An ultrasound scan may be performed to assess ovarian size and the presence of any pelvic and abdominal free fluid. If complications are suspected, the patient may require an arterial blood gas, chest x-ray, electrocardiogram and CT pulmonary angiography or ventilation/perfusion scan.

Although in most cases OHSS is self-limiting, these patients require supportive management and continuous monitoring. Hospital admission must be considered in women who are experiencing severe pain such that it cannot be managed in the community, who are unable to maintain adequate fluid intake, who don't adhere to treatment or follow-up, who have severe or critical OHSS or who are worsening despite outpatient management. The team in charge of the woman's fertility treatment should also be informed of her admission.

Table 94.1 Classification of ovarian hyperstimulation syndrome (OHSS)

Grade	Features
Mild OHSS	Abdominal bloating Mild abdominal pain Ovarian size < 8 cm³
Moderate OHSS	Moderate abdominal pain Nausea +/– vomiting Ultrasound evidence of ascites Ovarian size 8–12 cm³
Severe OHSS	Clinical ascites +/– pleural effusion Oliguria Haematocrit >45% Hyponatraemia Hypo-osmolality Hyperkalaemia Hypoproteinaemia Ovarian size > 12 cm³
Critical OHSS	Tense ascites/large pleural effusion Haematocrit >0.55 WCC >25,000/ml Oliguria/anuria Thromboembolism Acute respiratory distress syndrome

Appropriate analgesia and anti-emetics should be provided for these women, avoiding non-steroidal anti-inflammatory medications. Patients should be encouraged to drink to thirst to correct the intravascular dehydration, but in the acute phase, intravenous fluids may be needed for initial correction of the dehydration. Intravenous albumin may also be required to correct the hypoproteinaemia. Patients should be monitored with daily weights, blood tests, fluid balance and abdominal girth measurements to monitor progress. All patients admitted with OHSS must receive thromboprophylaxis with low molecular weight heparin and anti-embolic stockings. In most cases, mild pleural effusions spontaneously resolve with supportive management. Paracentesis should be considered in patients with tense and painful abdominal distension, shortness of breath or respiratory compromise and/or oliguria despite fluid replacement, all secondary to ascites.

This patient should be admitted for inpatient management of OHSS. Women and their partners should be counselled that the management is mainly supportive until it resolves spontaneously. For very unwell patients, a multidisciplinary team approach may be required in the intensive care setting to manage these patients appropriately.

 Key Points

- Suspect OHSS in patients with signs of fluid overload or ascites who are undergoing fertility treatment (IVF).
- Look carefully for signs of complications – pleural effusions, pericardial effusions, ascites and pulmonary emboli.
- Treatment is largely supportive with paracentesis, fluid monitoring, albumin replacement and venous thromboembolism prophylaxis.
- Very unwell patients should be monitored on the intensive care unit with multidisciplinary input.

History

A 35-year-old black lady comes into the Emergency Department feeling generally unwell. She is 30 weeks into her second pregnancy. She had a normal vaginal delivery with her first child 6 years ago. She has been suffering with a headache for the last 3 days, but today noticed that this has become significantly worse and that she has been seeing flashing lights. Over the last week, she had some mild epigastric pain, which she just put down to indigestion. She has also noticed that she has developed leg swelling in both legs over the past few weeks. Her blood pressure at booking was 115/65 mmHg.

Examination

On examination, her blood pressure is 170/101 mmHg and heart rate is 75 bpm. Her abdomen is soft but mildly tender in the epigastrium. The symphysiofundal height measures equal to dates. She has bilateral pitting oedema to mid-calves and hyper-reflexia is noted in the upper and lower limbs. Three beats of clonus were observed at both ankles. Her fundi appear normal when using the ophthalmoscope.

Investigations
• *Urinalysis:* 3+ protein, ketones negative, nitrites negative, leucocytes negative, glucose negative.

Questions

1. What is the likely diagnosis in this patient?
2. How would you go on to further investigate and manage her?

DISCUSSION

It is highly likely that this patient has pre-eclampsia and must be investigated and managed promptly. Pre-eclampsia is a multi-system disorder characterised by pregnancy-induced hypertension occurring after 20-week gestation and significant proteinuria. In severe cases, this can lead to eclampsia, defined as the occurrence of one or more convulsions on the background of pre-eclampsia. Severe pre-eclampsia and eclampsia are rare complications in pregnancy with 0.5% of maternities in the United Kingdom suffering from severe pre-eclampsia and 0.05% suffering from eclampsia. HELLP syndrome (haemolysis, elevated liver enzymes and low platelets) is an important and well-recognised complication of severe pre-eclampsia. Small-for-gestational-age babies and intrauterine growth restriction are common findings in 20%–25% of preterm and 14%–19% of term babies from mothers with pre-eclampsia, secondary to placental insufficiency. Risk factors for the development of pre-eclampsia include extremes of age, primigravida, multigravida with a new partner, previous history of pre-eclampsia, obesity and African ethnic origin.

Women with pre-eclampsia must have a raised blood pressure, which may be graded as mild, moderate or severe (Table 95.1), and significant proteinuria in the absence of a urinary tract infection.

Common features in the history include symptoms of severe headache, visual disturbances and epigastric pain with or without vomiting. When examining a patient with suspected pre-eclampsia, look for clonus, papilloedema, hyper-reflexia, oliguria and peripheral oedema. Some women may have no prodromal signs or symptoms.

It is important to distinguish pre-eclampsia from chronic hypertension, which existed prior to pregnancy. It is useful to look at the blood pressure at the time of booking to assess this and to check whether there was any protein in the urine at booking that may indicate underlying renal disease. Pre-eclampsia/eclampsia may also be confused with other diseases including antiphospholipid syndrome, thrombotic thrombocytopenic purpura (TTP), haemolytic uraemic syndrome (HUS) and primary epilepsy.

Measurement of blood pressure is a key part of assessing such patients; however, it is important to ensure that this is measured accurately. Remember that the cuff must be of the appropriate size and should be placed at the level of the heart to establish a baseline blood pressure. Serial blood pressures should be performed every 15 minutes until the patient is stabilised. Two plus of protein on the urine dipstick can be taken as significant proteinuria; however, this must be confirmed by a more accurate test including either a spot albumin:creatinine ratio ($\geq$30) or a 24-hour urine collection (>0.3 g in 24 hours). Blood tests including full blood count and liver function must be taken on these women to assess for HELLP syndrome. Close monitoring of renal function and fluid balance is also essential. In an acute setting, a fetus above 28 weeks gestation must be monitored with cardiotocography, and later a growth scan with foetal Dopplers should be arranged to assess for foetal wellbeing.

Table 95.1 **Grading of hypertension in pre-eclampsia**

Mild hypertension: Systolic 140–149 mmHg; diastolic 90–99 mmHg
Moderate hypertension: Systolic 150–159 mmHg; diastolic 100–109 mmHg
Severe hypertension: Systolic $\geq$160 mmHg; diastolic $\geq$110 mmHg

This patient has severe pre-eclampsia and must be treated urgently. Labetalol given either orally or intravenously is usually first line. Oral nifedipine and intravenous hydralazine can also be used for acute management. Atenolol, angiotension-converting-enzyme inhibitors and angiotension-receptor blockers should be avoided antenatally. Every trust should have its own stepwise protocol on the management of pre-eclampsia. Magnesium sulphate (4 g IV) is the drug of choice used to control seizures and also provides neuroprotection for the fetus if delivery seems imminent in fulminant pre-eclampsia. Fluid restriction is advised to reduce the risk of pulmonary oedema.

This patient will require urgent transfer to the High Dependency Unit or labour ward for stabilising and monitoring as she is at risk of an eclamptic fit. She will need admission until the blood pressure is stabilised and a maintenance regime has been established. In cases of uncontrollable blood pressure or eclampsia, delivery of the fetus via an emergency caesarean section may be required.

 Key Points

- Pre-eclampsia should be considered in all women in the third trimester with headache, elevated blood pressure or proteinuria.
- Perform serial blood pressure monitoring, urine analysis and blood tests to look for HELLP syndrome in the Emergency Department.
- Intravenous magnesium (4 g) is the first-line treatment for eclamptic seizures.
- In cases of uncontrollable pre-eclampsia or eclampsia, emergency caesarian section may be required.

CASE 96: BREATHLESSNESS IN PREGNANCY

History

A 30-year-old woman comes in to the Emergency Department complaining of shortness of breath. She is 29 weeks into her first pregnancy. She complains of breathlessness that came on suddenly during the early hours of the morning and has worsened throughout the day. It is associated with right-sided tight chest pain, which is worse on inspiration. She does not report any cough or haemoptysis. She has never experienced these symptoms before and has no significant past medical or surgical history. The baby has been moving around well and otherwise the pregnancy has been low-risk.

Examination

Vital signs: heart rate of 113 bpm, blood pressure of 89/55 mmHg, respiratory rate of 22 bpm, oxygen saturation of 91% on room air. She has a body mass index of 37 kg/m². There is equal chest expansion and the chest sounds clear all over. Heart sounds are normal with no additional sounds. There is no calf or ankle swelling.

 Investigations

- Hb 13.0, WCC 7.0, platelets 316, CRP 3.
- *Arterial blood gas (on room air):* pH 7.36, paO$_2$ 10.6, paCO$_2$ 5.9, HCO$_3^-$ 23.
- *Electrocardiogram:* Sinus tachycardia 110 bpm, evidence of 'S1, Q3, T3' pattern
- *Chest x-ray:* Normal

Questions

1. What is the diagnosis in this patient?
2. What further investigations are required in this woman?
3. How should she be managed?

DISCUSSION

This patient has a pulmonary embolism (PE). Venous thromboembolism (VTE) is still recognised as one of the leading direct causes of maternal death in the United Kingdom, although the number of reported fatalities following a PE has significantly reduced over the last few years. The overall prevalence of PE in pregnancy is between 2% and 6%. Pregnancy increases the risk of developing a venous thromboembolism by four to five times, compared to non-pregnant women of the same age. A total of 89% of women who died from a PE in the United Kingdom between 2006 and 2008 were found to have identifiable risk factors. It is therefore essential to risk-assess patients early at booking and during their antenatal care. Pre-existing risk factors for VTE include previous VTE, thrombophilia, age over 35 years, medical comorbidities, obesity, smoking, parity of 3 or more, dehydration and immobility. Pregnancy itself acts as a risk factor due to its hypercoagulable state.

Dyspnoea, pleuritic chest pain and haemoptysis may all be features of the history, although symptoms can be absent. Collapse and central chest pain may indicate a massive PE. On examination, the patient may have a raised respiratory rate, tachycardia and low oxygen saturations. She may have a raised jugular venous pressure and signs of a deep vein thrombosis in the leg.

Alternative diagnoses that should be considered include acute coronary syndrome, pneumonia, pneumothorax, sepsis, exacerbation of asthma or COPD and heart failure.

Blood tests should include an arterial blood gas, which classically shows respiratory alkalosis but may be normal with small PEs. A D-dimer should not be performed in pregnant patients with suspected VTE. Before commencing anticoagulant therapy, the patient's liver and renal function and coagulation profile should also be checked. An ECG must be performed to investigate for cardiac causes of symptoms and often shows sinus tachycardia with a PE. Evidence of right heart strain, right bundle branch block and the classic triad of 'S1, Q3, T3' can sometimes be seen. A chest radiograph must be performed in looking for other causes of symptoms. In women with signs and symptoms of a deep vein thrombosis (DVT), a compression duplex ultrasound of the legs should be considered. Diagnostic tests in the absence of features of a DVT are either a ventilation/perfusion (V/Q) lung scan or a computerised tomography pulmonary angiogram (CTPA). If the radiograph is abnormal and there is no indication of a DVT, a CTPA is the preferred imaging to investigate for a PE.

Patients must be assessed and stabilised in an 'ABCDE' approach. Treatment with low molecular weight heparin (LMWH) must be administered immediately for all pregnant patients with a suspected VTE, until a diagnosis is excluded, unless anticoagulation is strongly contraindicated. Warfarin is teratogenic and is contraindicated in the first trimester. Although safe beyond this, it is difficult to optimise, requires regular monitoring and can cause problems with excessive bleeding if not stopped early enough before delivery. Therefore, LMWH is the preferred treatment in pregnancy. Anticoagulation should be continued for the duration of the pregnancy and for at least 6 weeks postnatally, and at least 3 months of treatment should be given in total. LMWH or an oral anticoagulant can be given postnatally and warfarin is safe with breastfeeding.

As this patient is hypoxic and tachycardic, she should be admitted for investigation and management until her observations stabilise. The patient should be followed up regularly in antenatal clinic upon discharge and where possible should be seen in an obstetric medicine or joint obstetric haematology clinic postnatally. A collapsed and shocked patient with a massive PE must be managed in a multidisciplinary team of physicians, obstetricians, anaesthetists and radiologists.

Key Points

- The risks of pulmonary embolism are increased in pregnancy.
- D-dimer should not be performed in pregnant patients as it will be elevated.
- If PE is suspected, CTPA or V/Q scanning may be performed to confirm the diagnosis.
- LMWH is the preferred method of anticoagulation and must be given for a minimum of 3 months.

History

A 30-year-old lady is brought in to the Emergency Department by her husband. She is 10 days postpartum following a normal vaginal delivery and is complaining of a 2-day history of palpitations. She is not experiencing any chest pain, shortness of breath or cough. Her husband is worried as he says that she is behaving differently. He tells you that she has been quite withdrawn at home and tearful at times. Recently she has also been expressing worries that someone might come to take her baby away. She says she feels constantly anxious and has been unable to sleep for a week. She is fearful that something may happen to her baby. It was an unplanned pregnancy and the baby is being bottle-fed. She is normally fit and well and has no past medical history. Her brother is on treatment for schizophrenia.

Examination

She is afebrile with a regular heart rate of 75 bpm and blood pressure of 127/75 mmHg. She is saturating at 99% on room air. She appears thin and fatigued. She does not maintain eye contact and appears restless. The baby starts crying during the consultation and the mother is not responsive. She does not make any contact with the baby or make any attempt to calm him down.

Questions

1. What is the most likely diagnosis?
2. How should she be investigated?
3. How should she be managed and who should be involved in her care?

DISCUSSION

This woman is most likely suffering from postpartum psychosis. This is a severe episode of mental illness that begins in the days or weeks following delivery and is considered a psychiatric emergency. It is rare and affects 1–2 in 1000 women who have a baby. According to the Confidential Enquiries into Maternal Deaths, suicide in pregnancy and up to 1 year postpartum is the leading cause of maternal death in the United Kingdom. Contributing to this is the lack of recognition of high-risk patients, delayed diagnosis and failure to manage these patients appropriately. Many women may not have any risk factors; however, some may have a previous history of postpartum psychosis, a pre-existing psychotic illness or a family history of mental illness. Women with bipolar disorder are particularly at risk.

Symptoms may be very varied and can change and evolve rapidly. Women often have symptoms of depression or mania. Some may be anxious, agitated and irritable, and some may have difficulty sleeping. Women may be withdrawn or more talkative with loss of inhibitions and flight of ideas. There may be symptoms and signs of paranoia, delusions or hallucinations.

Postpartum psychosis should not be confused with postnatal blues (also known as 'baby blues'). This is characterised by mild mood changes, including fatigue, anxiety, depression, irritability and tearfulness, which often peaks around day 4 or 5 postnatally. It is usually self-limiting and is very common, occurring in around 50% of new mothers.

Postpartum depression occurs in around 10% of postnatal women and involves the normal symptoms of depression such as low mood, loss of interest, loss of appetite, insomnia and feelings of worthlessness or guilt. The symptoms of depression must be present daily for at least 2 weeks to make this diagnosis.

Anaemia and hypothyroidism are other causes of fatigue and low mood. Causes of palpitations must also be considered in this patient including cardiac arrhythmias, hyperthyroidism and panic disorder.

Blood tests including full blood count, electrolytes, thyroid function and magnesium should be performed to investigate for anaemia, thyroid dysfunction and electrolyte imbalance as a cause of palpitations. An electrocardiogram should also be performed in anyone complaining of palpitations.

This patient needs admission and immediate referral to the on-call psychiatrist for stabilisation with psychotropic medications or in some cases even sedation. The perinatal mental health midwife should also be informed of this patient's admission and will need to be involved her care. She will also need an urgent referral to the Mother and Baby Psychiatric Unit for further specialist assessment and management. The Obstetric Consultant in charge of this patient's care must be made aware of the case.

This is a psychiatric emergency. Accurate and timely diagnosis and management are essential to avoid harm to both the mother and the baby. For those with thoughts of harm to self or others who do not consent to treatment, involuntary admission and treatment under the Mental Health Act or Mental Capacity Act may be required. Urgent transfer to a Mother and Baby Unit will help provide the supervision and support that is required in such cases.

Key Points

- Postpartum psychosis is a psychiatric emergency.
- Assessment should be a thorough clinical examination and investigations to rule out organic causes.
- The patient may need admission and treatment under the Mental Health Act or Mental Capacity Act.
- Multidisciplinary assessment and treatment with obstetricians, midwives and mental health team are essential.

MEDICOLEGAL

CASE 98: CONSENTING A PATIENT IN THE ED

History

A 22-year-old man presents to the Emergency Department with left-sided pleuritic chest pain. He told the triage nurse that it came on suddenly last night, and this was the first time it has happened. He walked to the ED and his girlfriend is present. The triage nurse has performed some vital signs, prescribed simple analgesia and prioritised him for a chest radiograph. The patient is in the resuscitation room for review.

Examination

Vital signs are as follows: respiratory rate of 22/min, blood pressure of 125/65, O_2 saturation of 96% on air, temperature of 36.5°C.

The patient appears comfortable at rest and does not appear to be in distress. There are reduced breath sounds on the left side of the chest with hyper-resonance on percussion. The trachea is in the midline.

 Investigations
- A chest radiograph shows moderate left-sided pneumothorax without mediastinal shift with an inter-pleural distance (collapse) of 3 cm measured at the level of the hilum.

You assess him with your Registrar who has asked you to consent him for needle thoracentesis and to get the necessary kit ready. You have not performed this procedure before.

Questions
1. What is the management of the simple pneumothorax?
2. How are you going to consent this man and what is best practice?
3. How does informed consent guidance differ for persons under 18 years?

DISCUSSION

This man has a simple spontaneous pneumothorax that requires aspiration via an interpleural drain kit.

You have not performed this procedure before and you have been asked to take informed consent from this man in the absence of your supervising registrar – is this best practice? The General Medical Council has formal guidance on obtaining informed consent and outlines the responsibilities of the treating doctor. 'Informed consent' is a process of joint decision-making between the patient and the doctor. The guidance states that you should clearly explain the diagnosis and the options available for treatment to the patient. You should have a good working knowledge of the treatment options with the ability to explain potential risks, complications and the failure to achieve the desired end-point. Ideally, you should be able to perform the procedure or treatment option being offered to the patient.

The patient should be of sound mind, be able to retain this information long enough to arrive at a balanced decision and be able to communicate this. This is termed 'capacity' and encapsulated in the Mental Capacity Act (2005). When explaining risks, complications and outcomes, language should be in terms that the patient may understand. An independent native language interpreter should be used if necessary, and if the patient has any questions, these should be answered in full prior to the procedure.

Risks of a thoracentesis include the following: unable to locate space, discomfort, infection, bleeding, neurovascular injury, lung injury and the failure to reach the desired end-point (persistent pneumothorax, recurrence). You should also inform the patient that you may need to proceed to an intercostal drain and discuss this separately.

Consent may be *implied* (such as rolling up a sleeve for blood pressure measurement), *verbal* or *written*. In cases of minor intervention, implied or verbal consent usually suffices. This should be witnessed and documented in the patient record along with any discussions regarding risks and complications. Although it is infrequently done, best practice would be to obtain written consent for an elective needle thoracocentesis/proceed to intercostal drain. Some specialties and trusts have generated standardised patient consent forms for common procedures, and these should be used if available.

The legal process of capacity and consent to treatment in adolescents and children is different. In general, one needs to have the permission of their parent or those with parental responsibility for anyone under 18 years. The law assumes that the mother has parental responsibility, but this must be checked. In some circumstances, young persons can consent for themselves. For example, 16- and 17-year-olds are presumed by law to be able to consent to medical treatment. Refusal of treatment, however, may be overturned by the parent or court of law in certain circumstances. Also 14- and 15-year-olds may be able to demonstrate capacity to consent for medical treatment, independently of their parents via the 'Fraser guidelines'. This refers to case law whereby a child demonstrated capacity to consent for oral contraceptive pill treatment against the wishes of her parents. A young person must be able to demonstrate that they understand the proposed treatment, the pros and cons and alternatives in a balanced way and is then termed to be 'Gillick competent'. There is no lower limit to Gillick competence, although in children of 13 years and under, parental consent is usually sought for all treatment.

In terms of best practice, consent in all patients under 18 years should be taken jointly with the parents and the young person and in line with the principles outlined for adults. Consent for most procedures should be written and require the signature of the parent or legal guardian. Any additional discussions and decisions should be documented in the patient record.

In the rare circumstance that a parent or guardian cannot be contacted in a life-threatening emergency, the doctor may act in the patient's best interests. Most hospitals do have a 24-hour legal team that may be able to help with complex queries, and this should be escalated via senior medical staff as soon as possible.

Key Points
• Informed consent must be obtained prior to all medical procedures. • All patients should have a 'capacity' assessment performed. • In those under 18 years of age, parental consent is usually necessary. • In life-threatening emergencies, medical professionals are able to carry out interventions in the best interests of the patient.

History

A 6-year-old child was seen in the Emergency Department by a trainee doctor 3 days ago and has returned with ongoing wrist pain. He tells you he fell over whilst playing outside. He was brought to the Emergency Department by his mother, and a radiograph of the wrist was performed. They were told that the wrist was sprained and was discharged home with the advice to come back if the pain did not settle. He has been unable to write at school and his teachers have sent him home. His mother is very unhappy.

Examination

There is isolated pain over the distal radius with some associated soft tissue swelling. No clinical deformity is noted. Neurovascular examination is normal. There is full range of motion of the wrist and the hand, but flexion and extension are painful. The child cannot grip a pen without significant pain.

Investigations
• Upon review of the radiographs, there is an undisplaced torus fracture of the distal radius.

Questions

1. What are you going to explain to the child and his mother?
2. How are you going to manage the injury?
3. Are there any adverse outcomes?
4. What mechanisms exist to report this failure?

DISCUSSION

This patient has a missed fracture of the distal radius. Torus or 'buckle' fractures are sometimes missed, as radiographic findings may be subtle. On occasion, they may be visible as a 'kink' or bend in the cortex in one view only. Once identified, you should check the radiograph carefully to see if the injury extends to the growth plate and for any other associated injuries.

Your first steps should be to explain your findings to the patient and his mother. The General Medical Council's guidance on good medical practice states that you must put the patient at the centre of the consultation and your behaviour must encompass openness, safety, quality, communication, partnership and trust. Most parents are relieved when a diagnosis is reached and they have clear guidance on treatment and prognosis. In this case, the injury is managed non-operatively in either a splint, or more commonly in a plaster of Paris backslab with follow-up in fracture clinic. The limb is usually immobilised for 4–6 weeks and return to full function is expected in 8–12 weeks post-injury depending on the exact type of fracture.

The next question for most parents is why was the fracture missed and what can be done to prevent it from happening again? There is a no-blame culture in the NHS and incidents such as this are encouraged to be reported. The simplest and most direct way to do this is to inform the Consultant or senior doctor in the ED. The Consultant will also take on the responsibility for investigating the incident. Another important reporting tool is the incident reporting form (Datix). This is accessible from most NHS intranets and provides a mechanism for reporting almost any incident. Once completed, the form generates a report and is assigned to the most appropriate person for investigation, risk classification and review.

These mechanisms form an important part of the governance process for the ED and help maintain quality and safety. Once the form is assigned to an investigator, steps can be taken to unravel why this incident happened and steps put in place to stop it from happening again. Was it a case of simple error or does the attending doctor require additional training? Did the doctor review the images on a non-diagnostic small screen? In any case, no matter what the circumstances were, this system allows anonymity and empowers all members of the team to report any issues in the ED.

Most EDs have several safeguards already in place regarding radiographs with abnormal findings. Firstly, radiographers will place the words 'red dot' on immediately abnormal radiographs. This serves as an additional reminder to the attending practitioner that there is an abnormality present. It originates from when radiographs were printed and radiographers used to place a red sticker or 'red dot' on abnormal films. However, it should not be relied on as a sole indicator and queries escalated to senior medical staff in real time.

The other safety mechanism is at the reporting stage. With electronic systems, reporting radiologists and radiographers can check that appropriate follow-up or actions have been taken. In those that have been 'missed' or in which there is a query, a report is usually communicated to the senior ED team for review and action as appropriate. It is therefore essential that the most up-to-date demographics and contact telephone numbers are recorded for all patients attending the ED.

If the parent is still unhappy and wishes to make a formal complaint, then they should be put in touch with Patient Advisory and Liaison Services (PALS). They form an important bridge for the patient, parent and the staff involved, and their ability to listen and understand the patient or parent concerns helps to focus the investigative process and provide an outcome for all involved within formally agreed timelines.

Key Points

- The patient should always be placed at the centre of the consultation, and in cases of error, openness and probity are essential.
- The incident reporting form (Datix) provides a mechanism to report error or mistakes anonymously.
- Safeguards already exist in most Emergency Departments to ensure abnormal radiographs are acted upon.

History

A 90-year-old woman has been brought into the Emergency Department as a priority call. She has a suspected broken hip. Her carers have brought in her medication in a dosset box that includes metformin, gliclazide, bumetanide, aspirin and simvastatin. The carer is unsure when the medications were last given.

The attending doctor prescribes the following for hyperkalaemia: '50 mL 50% dextrose with 50 units actrapid iv, infuse over 15 minutes'. As the department is busy, the nurse asks the doctor to co-sign the infusion and starts the pump. The patient becomes unresponsive shortly after the infusion is started. A senior doctor is called and reviews the patient. The blood glucose is now 2.5 mmol/L. The infusion is stopped and the hypoglycaemia corrected. The patient recovers.

Examination

Vital signs: temperature of 34.8°C, blood pressure of 90/60, heart rate of 140 and regular, respiratory rate of 28, 94% O_2 saturation on air.

The patient is very frail and appears to be clinically dehydrated. Her left leg is shortened and externally rotated. Distal pulses are palpable in both legs.

Investigations
• A VBG performed on arrival shows the following: pH 7.10, pO_2 6.2, pCO_2 5.0, Na 148, K 7.0, Cl 110, glucose 4.7, lactate 4.0, HCO_3 16, BE −8.2
• An electrocardiogram (ECG) shows a sinus tachycardia with tall t-waves.

Questions

1. What has happened in this case?
2. What is your statutory obligation in terms of reporting?
3. What possible steps could be taken to prevent this from happening again?

DISCUSSION

This patient has suffered from iatrogenic hypoglycaemia due to an incorrectly prescribed insulin/dextrose infusion for hyperkalaemia. The assessing doctor correctly recognised that this patient was hyperkalaemic from an acute kidney injury and prescribed an insulin/dextrose infusion. The correct management for hyperkalaemia (K+ >6.5 mmol/L and or ECG changes) is as follows:

- Rehydration with 0.9% saline
- Calcium chloride or gluconate 10% 10 mL IV
- Nebulised salbutamol 5 mg
- 50% dextrose with 10 units of actrapid over 15–30 minutes with blood glucose monitoring every 10 minutes.

The adverse event arose from the prescription of the insulin, which was five times the recommended amount.

The case was referred up to the senior doctor and nurse in real time to review the patient, prevent further harm, support those involved (staff and patient) and gather information. All steps taken to correct or mitigate error should be documented in the patient record.

There is an ethical duty to inform the patient and their relatives of the event. 'Good Medical Practice' published by the GMC outlines the duties of a doctor. When an error occurs, there is a duty to inform the patient and their family as soon as it is practical, apologise and explain why it may have happened and the steps taken to mitigate this. There is also a statutory legal obligation known as the 'duty of candour'. This was introduced in 2014 and enshrined in the Health and Social Care Act. It applies to all adverse events that may cause 'significant harm' to the patient. There is no exhaustive list of events, but the National Patient Safety Agency (NPSA) provides guidance to identify them. The duty of candour is a legal extension of the ethical duties of a doctor to inform patients when things go wrong, and provides a framework for patients and relatives to get a transparent, accurate and truthful account of why things happened. As part of the duty of candour, all health care practitioners have an obligation to report error.

For this case, an incident form (Datix) should be filled out in real time. It should include a short narrative of what happened and steps taken to remedy the adverse incident as well as the details of the affected patient. If possible, the patient and their family should be informed of the event preferably by the duty senior doctor and nurse. The Datix form is then assigned to an appropriate senior person for investigation, review and risk-grading. Adverse events related to the prescription or administration of insulin are listed as 'never events' by the NPSA, and so this event will be subject to a formal serious incident (SI) investigation process. There is no fixed definition of a SI, but they represent serious systemic failure or events that may cause serious patient harm.

After the initial recognition of a potential SI, a report with a timeline narrative must be generated for review within 72 hours of reporting. A panel of senior experts will then ascertain if the event is of sufficient magnitude or system failure to proceed with a formal investigation. A lead investigator will be assigned and a multidisciplinary team will be created to perform a root cause analysis and generate a report. This case would require senior doctors, nurses and pharmacists as well as other staff who can help look at human factors and reasons for system failure. The culture promoted is not one of individual blame but to try and understand why the adverse incident happened and what can be done to prevent it.

Once the report is completed, it is imperative that themes and lessons learned are disseminated to the wider team, and it is an essential part of the governance process that ensures quality and safety in health care. In this case, potential human factors are identified: the ED environment was busy and the safety check of a second non-prescriber was negated. Often, these errors arise not because of single failure but because of multiple errors lining up – the 'swiss cheese model' whereby lots of 'holes' line up to allow adverse events to happen.

Potential mechanisms to prevent this event in the future could be to disallow prescriber checking for insulin infusions, pre-made infusions or protocolised prescribing via an electronic system or stickers/proforma. Decisions about change in process should be considered at a departmental governance meeting and involve pharmacists, nurses and clinicians together. The patient and family will be supported through the process via a dedicated liaison, and feedback and lessons learned should be shared with the family. Hospitals maintain central lists of known risks, and they form an important part of reducing patient harm.

It is essential that pastoral care is provided to the prescribing doctor and the administering nurse as considerable self-blame and doubt are often encountered by medical professionals in this position. Trusts do have formal procedures for support, and these should be activated to provide the necessary care. Other organisations such as the British Medical Association (BMA) may also be able to provide independent services.

 Key Points

- NHS trusts have a legal duty to report serious adverse events known as the 'duty of candour'.
- An initial investigation must be performed within 72 hours of reporting followed by a full root cause analysis investigation.
- Learning points and process change must be shared with the wider team to prevent recurrence.
- Both the affected patient and staff involved must be supported through the investigation process.

LABORATORY TEST NORMAL VALUES

Abbreviation		Normal Range and Units	
WCC	White cell count	$3.0–10.0 \times 10^9/L$	
Hb	Haemoglobin	13–17 g/dL	
MCV	Mean corpuscular volume	80–99 fL	
PLT	Platelet count	$150–400 \times 10^9/L$	
Neuts	Neutrophil count	$2.0–7.5 \times 10^9/L$	
Na	Sodium	135–145 mmol/L	
K	Potassium	3.5–5.1 mmol/L	
Ur	Urea	1.7–8.3 mmol/L	
Cr	Creatinine	66–112 mmol/L	
CRP	C-reactive protein	0–5.0 mg/L	
Bili	Bilirubin	0–20 µmol/L	
AST	Aspartate aminotransferase	10–40 IU/L	
ALT	Alanine transaminase	10–50 IU/L	
ALP	Alkaline phosphatase	40–129 IU/L	
ALB	Albumin	34–50 g/L	
TSH	Thyroid stimulating hormone	0.2–4.0 mIU/L	
T4	Levothyroxine	10–20 pmol/L	
		Arterial	**Venous**
pH	pH	7.35–7.45	7.31–7.41
pCO_2	Partial pressure carbon dioxide	4.7–6.0 kPa	5.5–6.8 kPa*
pO_2	Partial pressure oxygen	10.6–13.3 kPa	4.0–5.3 kPa*
HCO_3	Bicarbonate	22–28 mmol/L	
BE	Base excess	–2 to +2	
Lactate	Lactate	0.5–2.2 mmol/L	
Gluc	Glucose	4–8.0 mmol/L	

* To convert kPa to mmHg, divide by 0.133.

INDEX